REIKI

True Stories to Inspire You

By

Philip Westwood

AuthorHouse™ UK Ltd.
500 Avebury Boulevard
Central Milton Keynes, MK9 2BE
www.authorhouse.co.uk
Phone: 08001974150

First published by AuthorHouse 08/03/2011

ISBN: 978-1-4567-7494-3

Email: philipreiki@gmail.com
Website: www.reikiisphilipwestwood.co.uk

Any people depicted in stock imagery provided by Thinkstock are models,
and such images are being used for illustrative purposes only.
Certain stock imagery © Thinkstock.

This book is printed on acid-free paper.

authorHOUSE®

Contents

Chapter 6

Chapter 7

Chapter 8

Chapter 9

Foreword by Reiki Master Linda Prestidge

This book has been written for those who never cease to be amazed by the power of Reiki and for those who may not have yet experienced but are about to be amazed by the power of Reiki.

Reiki has been for many years now an essential part of my life as indeed it has become for Philip Westwood.

I have known Phil for many years. We met at a time when his wife Kim and I were working together at a salon. Phil and Kim also at this time owned and managed a woodland. It was during these years that I got to know Phil and became aware of how passionate he is about nature and the connection that all living things have. So it was no surprise to me when he expressed his desire to learn Reiki.

The following pages of this book will demonstrate to you the beauty and power of Reiki energy.

For those of you who know nothing at all about Reiki, I suggest you read with an open heart and a non-judgmental mind. For those that are familiar with Reiki, this book will reinforce that which you already know, and for those of you who are fortunate to know Phil and have been treated with Reiki by him and I include myself here, you will absolutely be sure that REIKI WORKS.

From time to time in our lives we find ourselves in need of help, and seemingly out of nowhere the answer comes. The answer came to me at such a time in the form of Reiki. First of all, I went for treatments, and then received the attunements up to Master Level. Sometime after this a friend had said to me, well now that you are attuned to Reiki you should never be ill again. The oversight on this belief is that illness or disease starts in the body, whereas it is now much more widely understood that illness/disease (dis-ease) in fact manifests in the body often from our inability to 'let go' of beliefs that we hold in our minds.

Through the use of Reiki we can discover how to return to a peaceful mind and healthy body.

Linda Prestidge

Introduction

This book is about my personal journey into the realms of Reiki healing with a fleeting glimpse of nature, because they are one. Whether we feel at one with nature or not, we *are* nature. We are all part of the intricate web of life; but unfortunately our need for natural resources has created a huge destructive imbalance on our planet that has initiated our on-going struggle for survival. As individuals, we may feel that it is not our responsibility to do anything to reverse this trend, but if we put our accumulated positive energy to the task in hand, we can all 'survive and thrive' and enjoy the miracle of our Planet.

I have spent more than twenty years working with, and for nature in one way or another and it has become apparent to me that what we send out to the Universe, we get back! If we tread gently, give more and take less, our world will be filled with joy and happiness.

A huge amount has been written on the subject of Reiki by some highly qualified practitioners with many years of experience, this book is a journal of some of *my* experiences and those of some of my clients and students.

I make no claims that Reiki can *cure* anything; I do however testify that the contents of this book are factual, truthful and correct and it is my wish that this publication will stir your imagination and open your mind to some remarkable possibilities. I have been very fortunate to witness some amazing healings over the years, but I feel that an element of trust is necessary if we are to believe in anything.

Some cultures have very little grounds for their faith and beliefs but their faith is un-movable, their truth is in their trust and the beliefs of their ancestors, parents and culture. Over thousands of years, that trust has been sorely tested but against all the odds, it still holds strong.

The point I am trying to make here is that sometimes we have no grounds to trust. We need to *see* these things with our own eyes and only then are we able to make a rational judgment. It is this *seeing* that limits our sensory awareness because we are meant to use all of our senses, not just our vision. Science has proved that many things are invisible to the naked eye but we now know that they exist, so why do we put so much trust in our eyes? Our other senses are equally as important but we rarely use them to their full potential, these extraordinary senses come into play when treating people with Reiki and they are essential because they enable us to respond to the ever changing flow of 'Life force energy.'

Acknowledgements

The past few years have been remarkable for me as a Reiki practitioner and teacher because I have discovered how Reiki brings life, health and happiness into our lives.

Reiki is pure and this is of great comfort to me as I walk my Reiki path to enlightenment.

I have met many people. Some were in need of Reiki for their physical problems while others felt that their needs were very little until they tried a treatment, and then Reiki gave them something very special, a new understanding of their world and insight that gave them freedom.

I would like to thank everyone that I treated in Cyprus because these clients were a constant reminder to me that Reiki brings people into our lives to be healed and for us to learn from the experience.

My students have taught me many things and the friendship that they gave me will remain in my heart forever. I am very fortunate because these students are now practicing and teaching Reiki and this has helped to raise the profile and standards of Reiki, I wish them success and happiness for the future.

My dear friend and Reiki teacher Linda is an inspiration to me, without her there would be no stories to tell and I thank her most sincerely for her help and support during my Reiki journey and for the remarkable insights that I have yet to experience.

I would also like to thank Ohn Mar and Mi Chaw for being so patient with Kim while she took the photographs for the book.

Ohn Mar has a very special place in my heart. Nothing was too much trouble for her and when I asked her if she would be willing to be a model for the photographs in the book she stayed up until the early hours of the morning because she wanted to make her own dress for the photographs! I shall treasure those photographs forever, what a shining light she is.

Sandra and Steve have supported me in many ways; they edited the book and helped me to put it into an order that made sense. Without their help and encouragement I would still be writing the book! Thank you both so much.

And my wife Kim, she needs a medal for her patience; she was a constant source of inspiration to me as I know It's not easy being the wife of someone who stays up late into the early hours and then works all day. Bless her, she is a treasure.

And finally, I met Cheryl and George Carter when I first arrived in Cyprus and they have become dear friends, we miss them both and they are always in our thoughts. That's the wonderful thing about true friendship; it stands the test of time.

The Reiki Phenomenon

Let me see if you can relate to some of my experiences.

I would like to start with a common phenomenon. How many times have you thought about someone you haven't spoken to for a while, and then a minute later your phone rings and it's him or her on the phone! What are the odds of this happening by chance? Here is a thought. Did your friend subconsciously sense your thoughts and decided to call you or was it the other way around; did you receive their thoughts first? Well, we may not be able to answer these questions, but one thing is for sure, most of the time we are not aware that we are *receiving or sending* anything at all because we have forgotten how to still our minds and thoughts because we are, for the most part, de-sensitized to our sensory capabilities.

Our senses do take control when necessary and here is another example. It relates to a mother's intuition. A mother may instinctively *know* that her child is in danger or has been injured because of what she is 'feeling,' she may call the school that her child attends only to be told that there has been an accident and her child has been injured.

The odds against this 'feeling' being correct statistically are huge, but it happens all the time and this is another example of how the human psyche can 'sense' or feel on a 'need to know basis.' If you put these theories to the test you may find some answers, but often, there are no logical answers to how these things are possible.

Science is amazing and without it we would still be in the Stone Age but there are many things that have not yet been proven scientifically and it is these areas of the unknown that we will benefit from when they are discovered in the future.

I have treated and trained a few students that were scientists, their perspectives and outlook on life are constantly being re-evaluated as they discover new things. 'Does Reiki really work'? Or 'do I have to believe in Reiki for it to work'? are frequently asked questions by some of these people.

I have had the opportunity to treat a number of sceptics over the years and a good percentage of these individuals ended up having experiences that changed their views and opinions, not only about Reiki but about other aspects of their lives. Unfortunately their doubts about what they believed has still left many un-answered questions.

As humans we have the brain capacity and limitless opportunities to develop our understanding of many things; all we really have to do is keep an *open mind* until we find an answer that we can trust and feel comfortable with.

Some people are what I would call *open sceptics*, they may be willing to try a Reiki treatment or even participate in a Reiki seminar, and this is because they are searching for factual proof that what they are being told is actually correct.

Then there are the *closed sceptics*. These individuals are not interested or willing to change their beliefs in the slightest way; their world is blinkered because it is restricted by their will, so which category do I fit into, sceptic or a believer in anything and everything? Well, I am still learning and the knowledge that comes with this is on-going, however, time has taught me to 'keep an open mind.' I don't believe or disbelieve in anything until I have proof one way or the other. Eventually through the test of time we will all have a better understanding of many things, including Reiki.

Chapter 1

COMPARISONS BETWEEN REIKI AND OTHER COMPLEMENTARY THERAPIES.

On occasions clients ask me if Reiki therapy works like other forms of complementary/alternative medicine; there are many therapies that can be combined with Reiki to benefit clients, here is a sample.

ACUPUNCTURE

If you make a comparison between Reiki, Acupuncture or Reflexology you need to be aware that they have little in common with regard to the way that they work, but they all have some benefits to offer.

For example, with acupuncture, the therapist may spend an hour or so filling in a lengthy lifestyle questionnaire with you, this should give the practitioner an overview of your needs and also provide some indications or reasons for any imbalances that you may have or show symptoms of.

The practitioner will then make a diagnosis and then insert the needles to restore the balance in those parts of the body that require them. Conscious thoughts, logic and reasoning were used to come to a diagnostic conclusion before the treatment could begin.

REFLEXOLOGY

A Reflexology treatment is done predominantly on the feet and sometimes on the hands. The reflexologist *feels* for the imbalances on the energy zones on various parts of the feet with his or her hands. These zones on the hands and feet relate to the reflex areas that correspond to all of the major organs, glands and body parts.

The feet are extremely sensitive and the therapist will systematically work on these zones, *feeling* for any abnormalities or imbalances. The 'feeling' that I am talking about here is from the therapists' *sense of touch*. A practitioner should never make a diagnosis during or after the treatment unless he or she is medically qualified to do so and if any imbalance is found, the practitioner will apply pressure on these areas to help to alleviate the problem. In this instance, a combination of touch and conscious thoughts was used to determine which parts of the body needed balancing.

With either of the above therapies, Reiki can be used to enhance the treatment so if you practice Reflexology, Acupuncture and Reiki, a better balance will be achieved because the patient will invariably *take* Reiki at the same time whether you are treating them with it or not!

REIKI

Before starting a Reiki treatment, the therapist should ask you a number of questions. The reason for asking these questions is to ascertain if you are taking any medication, suffering from stress or to find out if there are any contraindications that may prevent you from having the treatment. A Reiki practitioner with experience should also be able to recognize the names of common drugs that are frequently prescribed and mentioned during this consultation such as Insulin for Diabetics or Thyroxin for thyroid imbalance etc. The practitioner needs to be aware of any medical conditions that you are suffering from as they may well give some indication of your health on the day of the treatment.

I cannot stress enough that a diagnosis should never be given during or after a Reiki treatment unless the practitioner is medically qualified to do so and if you are taking prescription drugs on a regular basis you should inform your doctor that you are receiving Reiki treatments. This is because some medical conditions will improve after only one treatment and the need to take your medication may have to be re-assessed by your Doctor.

There is something else that should be taken into consideration before you have a Reiki treatment. When you have a treatment you are not being given Reiki by the therapist; Reiki is being 'taken by you.'

We have energy centres called 'Chakras' and they are responsible for taking what is needed from the practitioner so whenever you come into contact with a Reiki source, your chakras will automatically take what they need unless your conscious thoughts decide not too, this is your free will at work.

We sometimes *think* that we know what is best for us, fortunately our Chakras *know* what is best for us and have the ability to override our thoughts when necessary, this enables the chakras to take exactly what we need. I would like to give you an example of how your Chakras do this.

Chapter 2

Is a Reiki treatment of benefit to everyone?

In my work I spend some of my time waiting for clients to arrive for their treatments; this 'waiting time' is often in a Spa reception area and I am frequently the only person sitting there. And when a guest arrives, Reiki energy starts to flow automatically from my hands without any conscious thoughts from myself. The guest who may be sitting on the other side of the room may be oblivious to the fact that I am a Reiki Master, but may be in need and their energy centres will open to take Reiki from the nearest source, and that source is me. Occasionally a guest will begin to cry and from experience I now understand why this happens. It is because this individual has been unable to let go of an emotional issue or problem themselves and the energy that their chakras take while sitting there goes directly to the cause of the problem to release it. The reality is that Reiki didn't make this person cry, it enabled them to cry and it gave them an emotional freedom that they couldn't give themselves.

Reiki can't work against your higher self or best interests and quite often it appears that a Reiki treatment has been of no benefit at all to an individual. An example of this is when someone appears to enjoy telling others how unwell they are, it is as if they are *happy* to be ill. They allow their illnesses to feed off them and if they were to become well again, this would give them nothing to talk about and their illness would no longer be a dominating factor in their life. Under these circumstances their *will* has decided to hold on to the illness and this interferes with the body's ability to heal and balance itself, it is unfortunate that our *will* can prevent us from taking Reiki and leading a normal healthy life!

On the other hand, if *you* hated every minute of your illness and you were to have a Reiki treatment, the chances are that you would notice some improvement in your condition after just one treatment. This is because *you* hardly ever talk about your illness and don't want to give it space in your life; you would do anything to be fit and healthy!

I don't want to confuse you into thinking that all of our illnesses are psychosomatic because if that were the case we would all need to visit a psychiatrist to get help but what I am saying is that some of us become what we think and the more time and energy we spend worrying about something, the greater the risk we have of developing a physical symptom or condition. Show me someone who is suffering from I.B.S. (Irritable bowel syndrome) who is not also suffering from stress!

Our bodies react to stress in different ways, some of us enjoy a little stress while other cannot tolerate even the smallest amounts, and it is our individual sensitivity that sets us apart from each other, emotionally, physically and spiritually.

During a Reiki treatment Reiki energy goes directly to the cause of the problem; the treatment may not reduce the physical discomfort of the condition until the cause has been addressed and Reiki is able to differentiate between the cause, and the physical manifestation of the symptom, and to do this Reiki must have its own intelligence.

When I first heard this statement a few years ago, I didn't really understand or believe that this was possible, but after several thousand treatments, I now know it to be the case.

On many occasions, I would start a treatment only to be interrupted by the client who would ask me how I knew where their problem was, this was because as soon as Reiki was channelled, it travelled directly to the problem area in the body, and my client could feel it. At the start of a treatment the Brow or "Third Eye" is usually the first hand placement and on numerous occasions clients would tell me that his or her *knee* had begun to tingle or heat up. Invariably, this was where their worst problem was although my hands were nowhere near their knee, this indicates that Reiki knew where the problem was and travelled straight to it! After practicing for a number of years, Reiki has given me the confidence to let this 'intelligent energy' find and deal with the problems wherever they are located in the body.

IMPORTANT NOTE

Some of the technical information and techniques in this book can be found in various publications and of course on the Internet. The author and publisher assume no liability whatsoever for damages of any kind that occur directly from the application or use of the statements and techniques that are described in this book.

Reiki therapy should not be used as a substitute for conventional medical treatments; however it can be used to compliment them.

WHAT IS REIKI?

Reiki is a natural healing spiritual energy that is now practiced throughout many countries of the world. It is a system of natural healing that can bring positive benefits to those who have treatments or practice it. By the time you have read this book, you may have a very different opinion and hopefully a better understanding of what Reiki is and I have purposely kept this paragraph of the book brief because there are many ways to define what Reiki is. I would suggest that you make up your own mind for now. Your opinions may be totally different to mine because they may be based on your experiences of having treatments, or training or from what you have read or heard about Reiki elsewhere.

Chapter 3

THE ORIGINS OF REIKI

In 1551, Toshitane Chiba, a famous Samurai warlord attacked and conquered a city called Usui, the consequence of this was that the Chiba family took on the Usui name and this was common practice at the time. It was thought that Mikao Usui discovered Reiki around 1922, but there is now evidence that contradicts this; Mikao Usui may have been practicing Reiki a decade before this time.

Mikao Usui was born on the 15th August 1865 in the village of Taniai in the Yamagota County of the Gifu prefecture in Japan, in later life he became a lay Tendai priest called a Zaiki.

Usui sensei was born into a society based on the class system; his family were Hatamoto Samurai and were highly respected in the ranks of the Samurai. Unfortunately, from the 1860's onwards the Samurai were no longer needed and they were offered positions as public servants. The Samurai struggled to retain their identity as warriors and this was the beginning of the end for the Samurai class, forcing some of them to become outcasts and many of them became outlaws!

THE MEANING OR DEFINITION OF THE WORD REIKI

The two Kanji or pictograms that were used for the word "Reiki" were very common in Japan and were also used to describe other things that are not related to the word Reiki as we know it today. Only when Reiki came to the west was it given this title. We in the west translated the word to mean "Universal Life force Energy," Mikao Usui's translation would have been different and it may have had a spiritual connotation to it, such as 'Spiritual Energy.' You could also use the word Ki or Chi to demonstrate the flow of 'Life force energy' in and around the body and this would also be applicable.

We in the West sometimes translate the word 'Reiki' to mean 'Life force Energy' or 'Universal Life force Energy,' Mikao Usui described this life force energy as; 'The Spiritual energy to cure all ills.'

What is a Reiki treatment?

A Reiki treatment can be a five minute session for something such as a headache or last two hours or more. Generally, a professional treatment should consist of a one to one and a half hour session and the time spent on the treatment will depend on the needs of the client or patient and their time constraints.

A treatment consists of a series of hand placements, done with one or two hands at a time, or with one, two or more fingers which are placed on or over the energy centres of the body, these energy centres are called 'Chakras.' It is also possible to use the eyes and breath to channel Reiki into the body and to send Reiki distantly with the use of sacred Reiki symbols.

People have described to me what they thought a Reiki treatment was, but most of their interpretations were a long way short of the facts so I would suggest that if you are having a treatment for the first time, don't ask the practitioner what it will feel like! This is because if you are told what the common sensations are and then experience them, you may never know if those experiences were yours, or the words that were placed in your subconscious mind by the practitioner.

I always ask my clients if they have had a treatment before, and if the answer is no, I briefly explain about the hand placements etc. and allow them to have their own experiences. If they have had a treatment before I will ask them to relax and make themselves comfortable and let Reiki find any imbalance.

It is vital that the practitioner completes a pre-treatment consultation before the treatment begins and a post-treatment analysis at the end of the session; this is because the client may have a number of questions to ask you about his or her treatment and may want to ask or tell you about some of the other weird and wonderful things they may have experienced during their treatment.

Over the past few years it has been possible to access new techniques and information from Japan that were not readily available to practitioners before; for instance, I mentioned earlier that Reiki can flow from the breath, the eyes and other areas of the body at will. Some practitioners will be well versed with the use of these 'New' techniques. In fact, Mikao Usui developed these techniques many years ago, but we have only recently had access to them via the internet and through various publications. I strongly recommend that you seek out a practitioner who uses some if not all of these techniques and experience a treatment with them because these techniques can be very powerful and you may experience some sensations that you have never felt before from your own practitioner.

What does a treatment feel like?

When you have a treatment there are many sensations that you may feel. These range from the hot or cold hands of the practitioner, to tingling sensations almost anywhere in the body. Another common sensation is that of being pulled or pushed from a kind of magnetic energy or the feeling of something like static electricity flowing around or through your body. Clients also report that they feel very heavy, or as light as a feather when they are lying on the Reiki table. It is also common to *see* things during a Reiki treatment when your eyes are closed. I know what you are thinking, is this possible? Well, most of us are able to see when our eyes are closed, for example when we are 'sun bathing' we see the sunlight that is shining on our eyelids. This sometimes gives us the impression of seeing orange or yellow light and this is a reaction to the Sunlight shining through our eyelids. If you place your hands over your eyes this will limit the light reaching our eyelids and this gives us the impression that it is darker, but during a Reiki treatment sometimes the opposite happens. If the practitioner places their hands over your eyes you may experience a bright light or bright colours and this is in total contrast to what would happen if you did this to yourself.

Clients may also twitch, jump, laugh, cry, fall into a heavy sleep or may have an out of body experience and on rare occasions physically levitate off the couch! As you can see, the range of sensations and experiences that you may have may well be linked to your physical, emotional and spiritual needs and can be extremely variable.

I am intrigued by the reactions that people have to their Reiki treatments, some are 'blown away' by their experiences while others just fall into a peaceful asleep. I have learnt to let go of wanting to 'fix' or 'cure' everyone because I am not in charge of the healing. It is up to the client to take what is needed for their own wellbeing although it is a good idea to ask a client what benefits they would like to get from the session, this gives the practitioner some indication of the client's intent and can also help the client to be realistic about their expectations.

HOW OFTEN DO I NEED A TREATMENT?

This is the top question that clients ask me after having a treatment. It may take a day or two before you know what the benefits of your treatment are and I always recommend that you should wait a couple of days after your treatment to determine how you feel. You also need to take into account what your needs are before you decide if another treatment would benefit you.

It would be easy to tell everyone that only a course of treatments would make a difference to their health and well-being, but the fact is that sometimes one treatment is enough. If a practitioner tells you that a course of ex- number of treatments would be beneficial, question the motives for this advice and wait to see how you feel after the first treatment before you decide to invest in other sessions, remember, it is your body and who knows it better than you!

After having a treatment, you may feel really good so don't think that if you have another one a few days later that it will make you feel even better because in truth, this may not be the case. Another thing that is worthwhile doing is for you to try a treatment with a different practitioner from time to time; this will help you to check out the range and diverse nature of the treatments that you receive and eventually you will find a balance between being comfortable with the practitioner and receiving the best possible benefits.

WHAT ARE THE BENEFITS OF HAVING A TREATMENT?

The list of benefits that you may receive is limitless but if I had to make a generalization, I would say that Reiki may improve your wellbeing and health in one way or another. Sometimes a treatment can be a life changing event, especially if you have a chronic or long-term condition. The nature of the problem can sometimes be caused by something emotional such as a past traumatic event and having a Reiki treatment can be an excellent way of relieving the symptoms that may be linked to your emotional state. The cost of a treatment will vary from one practitioner to another and obviously if you are having a treatment in a 5 star Spa or a private practice in an amazing location you would expect to pay more than if you were having a treatment in someone's home. You should also be aware that if the treatment is not up to your expectations you should try another practitioner because the treatment and outcome may be much better next time.

A fair analogy of a Reiki treatment is that it is like having a meal in a restaurant, sometimes the service is poor and the meal mediocre and on other occasions it can be an amazing experience that you will never forget and will want to repeat again and again.

Chapter 4

HOW DO I FIND A COMPETENT PRACTITIONER OR MASTER?

You should start with a recommendation if you know of someone who has tried a treatment, or surf the Internet and look for organizations that specialize in Reiki.

When you find a practitioner that sounds promising, a few relevant questions will help you to decide whether you should book a treatment or not.

"How long have you been practicing Reiki" would be a good question to ask then add to this by asking if the person does any other kind of treatments? Personally, I would recommend that you choose a practitioner or 'Master' who specializes in Reiki because this shows a commitment to the profession. If, for instance you choose someone who does other treatments in addition to Reiki, how will you know much Reiki this practitioner does compared to these other therapies?

Another point to remember here is that a full-time 'working' Reiki Master should be doing lots of treatments and ideally be teaching.

There are many Masters who do not teach or treat clients and if you have asked the questions then you should opt for someone who is busy doing lots of treatments and teaching others. Another question that I am frequently asked is 'What is the difference between a practitioner and a Master? One might assume that the 'Master' would know more about Reiki than a practitioner and be a better option, but this may not always be the case!

Here is an example. A practitioner who specializes in Reiki and works five days a week doing treatments should be very experienced and will be an excellent channel for Reiki energy. A Master on the other hand who does hardly any treatments will not be such a good channel for this powerful energy and under these circumstances I would opt for the practitioner to give me a treatment, not the Master.

From these comments, you can clearly see that it is important to ask some relevant questions if you want to find a practitioner or Master that you can feel comfortable with and one that is right for your needs. When you have had a few treatments you may want to find a Master to teach you Reiki.

I would recommend that you meet your intended teacher face to face to see how you feel about him or her before you decide to register for a course. You may feel very relaxed in their company and this is a good indication, but if you feel a little uncomfortable then this might not be the right time or person to teach you.

You may want to study Reiki with a friend or colleague from work and if this is the case, give this some consideration as it will be more enjoyable for you both, and you can practice on each other while you learn.

WHAT IS A REIKI ATTUNEMENT?

A Reiki Attunement is an essential part of the Reiki training. The process is very unusual and personally, I can't think of anything that compares with the experience as it can be a profound, life-changing event.

There are three courses in the Usui system of natural healing. Some Masters will teach Level 1 and 2 together in a weekend and the Master-teacher course over the next few days and by the end of the week you can be a certified Reiki Master- Teacher! Fast tracking like this has created something of a dilemma because if it is so quick and easy to gain a Reiki certification, how effective can the treatments and training be and I have been told on many occasions that Reiki can't be any good because anyone can be a Reiki Master after a few days training!

Every Master has their own way of teaching and it's fair to say that most have very high standards; the way I look at this is that we have an obligation to our students. They are 'The future of Reiki' and it takes time and practice to learn the art. The majority of Masters that I know are trying to raise the standards of Reiki and this will undoubtedly improve the quality of the treatments and training and raise the profile of Reiki therapy in the future.

The Reiki attunements are seen as a secret initiation by some Masters, never to be shown to anyone unless they are part of the Master/Teacher training and only then are the students shown how to attune others to the Reiki source. Unfortunately, I think that when we try to maintain a veil of secrecy about something, we create more interest; this may be because we are intrigued, or because we wish to find out more about the unknown.

It must be said that attuning others to Reiki is very rewarding and there are occasions when I will 'give' an attunement to someone who is in need of it. One of these occasions is when someone is terminally ill and having an attunement will help the individual with the transition from this world to the next, the attunement will not however speed up the process of dying; it will merely allow the sick individual to have an easier passage.

An attunement is a sacred spiritual initiation that connects the student to a higher form of vibrational energy, this higher vibration heals and balances the Chakra system and connects the student, to become a channel for others.

Anyone can learn Reiki and anyone can become a Reiki Master, the ability to heal comes from the energy that is channelled from the Reiki Master when combined with the Reiki symbols and the Mantra's of these symbols and there are numerous ways to attune you to this energy, it can be from a hands-on experience and it can also be sent as a 'Distant attunement.'

SOME PHOTOGRAPHS OF THE ATTUNEMENT PROCESS

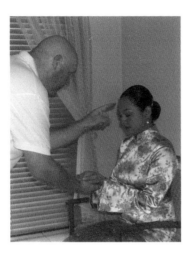 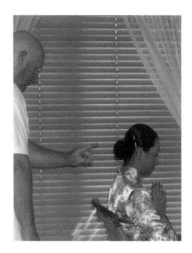

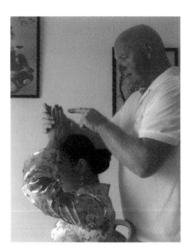

Personally, I prefer to do the attunements in the conventional way. I have a minimum of two students on the course because this helps them to have hands on experience and share from each other. Some Reiki organizations require proof of your training before they will include you on their list of working practitioners or teachers. I personally do not recognize a Reiki qualification if it has been done as a distant attunement without direct contact in the conventional way from a qualified Reiki Master.

Chapter 5

THE USUI-TIBETAN WESTERN STYLE OF REIKI

I am only going to explain the form or style of Reiki that I was attuned to here as there are many variations and a wealth of books published on the subject. Some of these books may show how the attunements are done while others will definitely not; this is because the symbols that are used during the attunement are sacred and should always be treated with great respect. Almost everyone has access to the internet now and the symbols can be found on a number of web-sites and numerous publications show some, if not all of the symbols that are in use today. Personally, I feel that there is no problem with having access to the symbols because being able to draw and memorize them is not enough to activate the energies that enable them to work. Only a Reiki Master-Teacher is able to attune others with the sacred initiations-attunements; and it is this that gives the student the energetic connection to channel 'Life force energy' into themselves and others.

SHODEN

When I was attuned by my Reiki Master Linda I was taught Usui-Tibetan Reiki, a western form. The first level is referred to as Reiki 1, First Degree, Level 1 and the Japanese call it 'Shoden,' meaning 'First Teachings.' In this form of Reiki there are 4 separate attunements in the first course and some Masters teach this course over a day or a week-end.

OKUDEN

The second level may be referred to as the Second Degree, Reiki 2 or the practitioner level and the Japanese call it 'Okuden' which means 'Inner Teachings.' This course can also be taught over a day or a week-end.

SHINPIDEN

The final level is sometimes called Reiki 3, the Third Degree or Master-Teacher level and the Japanese call it 'Shinpiden' meaning Mystery Teachings. This course is combined with A.R.T. – Advanced Reiki Training and I prefer to do this course over 5 days with a minimum of 30 hours teaching, other masters may teach this over a longer or shorter period of time.

SOME EXAMPLES OF OTHER FORMS OR STYLES OF REIKI

There are many other forms of Reiki, possibly over a hundred and as many organizations linked to them. Here are just a few examples:

Usui Reiki, Tibetan, Rainbow, Karuna, Raku Kei and Reiki Jin Kei Do etc.

With this wealth of information, how do you decide which is the right form of Reiki for you? Well, I recommend that you spend some time before you decide, Mikao Usui was the founder of the original form when he discovered Reiki in Japan, he developed the system of natural healing we call Reiki today and this would be a good place for you to start from. The internet will reveal a huge amount of information about Reiki but don't get too bogged down with the reading material because it can be confusing and there is no guarantee that the information will be factually correct.

You can also look for other likeminded people who are interested in Reiki. You may sometimes see practitioners advertising 'Reiki shares,' this term is used to describe those who come together to share their Reiki experiences and if you participate in a Reiki share you may have the opportunity to try a treatment from a number of hands placed on you at the same time! This will probably only last a few minutes for each person in the group but it is a wonderful way to experience the flow of Reiki energy for the first time and you can also ask the other participants at the meeting about their experiences of working with 'Life force energy.'

BYOSEN REIKAN-HO

Byosen Reikan Ho is a Japanese technique that is used for sensing imbalances in the body with your hands. Byosen Reikan literally means energy sensation of sickness, imbalance and disease. Byo means "disease, sickness" and Sen means "before, ahead, previous, future, precedence", "Rei means energy, soul or spirit" and Kan means emotion, feeling, sensation." This is an original technique from Usui Sensi which can be done on yourself or others.

Hand positions for practicing Byosen Reikan Ho (BODY SCANNING)

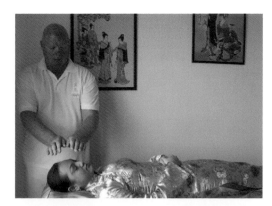 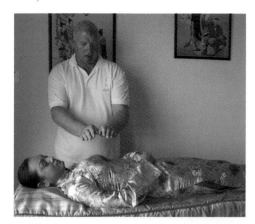

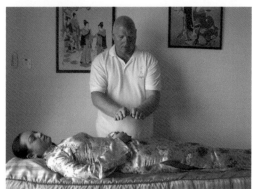 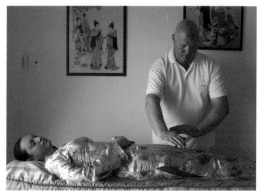

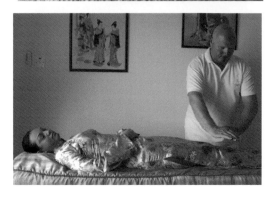 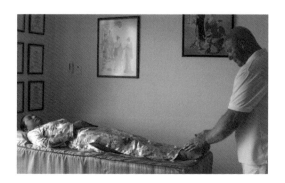

SOME OF THE ORIGINAL HAND POSITIONS TAUGHT BY MIKAO USUI

Treating the Crown

The Solar Plexus

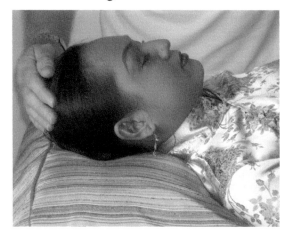

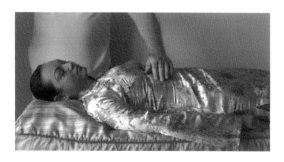

The Tanden or Hara

The Third eye

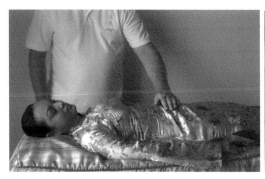

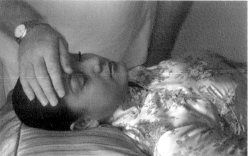

Mikao Usui used his intuition when treating patients and many of his hand positions incorporated the use of single or multiple fingers, one or both hands or the eyes and breath. Intuition is part of our sensory awareness and it can be developed with time and practice and using these techniques can make a huge difference to the outcome of a treatment.

AUTHOR'S BIOGRAPHY

I was born in a town called Smethwick in the heart of the industrial west-midlands and came from a working class family. I was the youngest of three children. My father worked as a labourer in a local foundry and my mother was employed in a factory assembling components for a cycle manufacturer.

As a young boy my life was happy and full of adventure, but I was a dreamer! One of my favourite pastimes was going to our local park with my friends where we would play on the swings, kick a football or fish for sticklebacks in the park pool. In those days the summers seemed to last forever and I always stayed out late until my mum called me in for supper and even then I would complain and cry because I wanted to stay out longer.

From the time I opened my eyes at first light, I would rush to go outside and play. I felt free when I was in the fresh air, even in inclement weather and it didn't matter to me what the weather was doing because there was always something that I could get up to. My problem was that I was always getting into trouble. There was no malice in me, but trouble was always just around the corner and if someone had been up to mischief, that someone was probably me! Looking back now, it was a miracle that my mum had the strength to rear me because she worked long hours in the factory and then more looking after me and my older brother and sister and it must have been exhausting for her.

When I was eight years old my Uncle Frank and Aunt Sally offered to take me fishing and *they* had a camper van! I had never been in a car before and I remember being unable to sleep because I was thinking about how wonderful the next day was going to be because I was going on a great adventure!

The next morning we set off to travel to Bewdley, a small market town on the banks of the river Severn. When we arrived my uncle set me up with a fishing rod and some strange wriggly things called maggots and what an amazing day it turned out to be because not only did I catch some fish; I saw horses, sheep and cows in the fields. This was a truly wonderful experience for me because where I lived in Smethwick, the only animals that I had seen were sparrows, pigeons and the occasional horse and cart that delivered our coal!

Later that evening on the journey home, I fell fast asleep on the back seat of the car, I was exhausted but very happy and what an adventure it had been. This had been an amazing day for me and I decided there and then that I wanted to live in Bewdley!

That summer flew by, and soon it was time to return to school, something I was not looking forward to. You see, I was very different from my school mates because *they* seemed to like going to school, I on the other hand felt like a caged animal, and if the truth be known, I think I was something of a feral child!

My older brother Terry and sister Jacky were more focused on getting an education to give them better career opportunities than me and they both passed their eleven plus examinations and went on to go to grammar school. I didn't have time for school, I used to go, but I always wanted to be somewhere else. On reflection, I did have a brain, but it was always being distracted by thoughts of fun and adventure! My mother despaired; and inevitably I failed my eleven plus examinations and had little or no interest in my future prospects, especially if that meant doing homework because I couldn't see the point of it all?

The inevitable happened and at the age of fifteen I left school with no formal qualifications but I did have a job to go to and 2 days later i started work as an apprentice Butcher! Over the next twenty years I drifted from one occupation to another and I tried many things. I took a job as a labourer on a building site, then a landscape gardener, a painter and decorator and a tool setter and it was while I was working in a factory that I had my first break, or to put it another way, a slipped disc!

I had to undergo surgery and it was during my recovery from the operation that I became interested in wildlife photography.

I had always been fascinated with wildlife as a child and while I was recuperating, I took some photographs of the wildlife near my home and for the first time in my life I found something that I felt comfortable with and was good at. I loved every minute of being at one with nature and I spent hours stalking Deer and Badgers in my local country park, but it took me another six months before I had a photograph of a Badger that I was satisfied with.

Badgers foraging for food

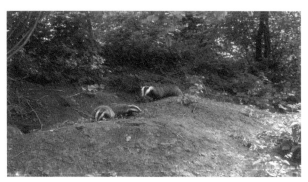

After a few months my spine healed and I started to look for work. I read about a vacancy for a schools liaison officer for an urban wildlife trust and immediately sent off for an application form and job description.

After completing the form there were several blank spaces when it came to the education – qualifications section but I didn't let that deter me because it looked like the job description had been written for me as everything on it was what I wanted and could do. I knew that I could communicate with others and be enthusiastic without any effort on my part and I thought that if I could just get an interview I might be able to talk my way into the post, a week later I was invited to attend an interview, I must admit that I was a little nervous but thought that this was just the opportunity I was waiting for. There were three people on the interview panel and I immediately felt a connection with them, this was until I was asked the question, "why did you apply for the position because you don't have the teaching qualification we asked for do you"?

I took a few seconds to compose myself then I said calmly, "When I read the job description, I thought that it had been written for me, every detail in it seemed to say it's me they are looking for."

My comments made everyone laugh, even I had a grin on my face and at that moment any nerves that I had, disappeared and I sailed through the remainder of the interview. I answered every question that was put to me with an air of confidence that surprised even me!

Later that evening my phone rang, it was the trust offering *me* the post! This was a wonderful feeling and a boost to my confidence and the following week I started work for the trust.

The post was only 30 hours per week, part-time and a one-off- six month contract but it was paid work and very rewarding and everyone who I came into contact with made me feel very welcome.

A few weeks before my contract ended, I started looking for another job; I liked the idea of working in a Country Park and the nearest one, 'Woodgate Valley Country Park' was not too far from where I lived, but unfortunately there were no vacancies. Undeterred; I enquired about voluntary work, logic told me that if I was willing to work for nothing now, I might be able to find paid employment there in the future and I would gain lots of valuable experience along the way.

I was offered work as a volunteer Ranger and worked every weekend for a year with the other staff taking children and adults on guided walks etc. My voluntary work eventually paid off and the post of Assistant Countryside Ranger was advertised. As I looked through the job description I noticed that one of the academic requirements was that I had to have an environmental Degree to apply, the problem was that all I had was a clean driving license and one year's experience of working with nature! Undeterred, I felt that what I lacked in academic qualifications, I could make up for with practical experience and my love of the countryside and fortunately this was enough to secure me the position.

It was at this point in my life that I met Kim, my wife. We were introduced to each other at a New Year's Eve fancy dress party by my friend Gloria; I was dressed as a confederate officer and Kim as an Indian squaw. It was some weeks later that I discovered that Gloria had been 'matchmaking' and knew Kim! She told us both what clothes we should wear to the party knowing that an Indian Squaw and a Confederate officer might find something in common to talk about, especially as she was going to introduce us to each other and she was right, six months later we were married!

ANOTHER EXCITING CHALLENGE

After several years, the role of my job as a Countryside Ranger had changed and I was now spending more of my time trying to prevent crime and vandalism instead of creating wildlife habitats and teaching people about nature conservation and I began to feel like a policeman!

Kim and I decided that it was time to take some initiative and after considering our options, we put our house on the market; I then applied for voluntary redundancy and started to search for a piece of broadleaved woodland because I had always dreamt of owning my own piece of woodland.

A year later we sold our house and purchased ten acres of ancient oak woodland called 'Grove Covert,' we re- named it 'Crown East Heritage Woodland' after the village that it was in. The wood was a couple of miles from the beautiful Cathedral city of Worcester in the stunning Worcestershire countryside. It took another nine months before things fell into place at work and then I was offered voluntary redundancy by Birmingham city council. My career as a Countryside Ranger had lasted 11 years and during this time I had been promoted to the position of Ranger. A month later I started work in our wood which was very neglected, but had a lot of potential but was in need of some tender loving care.

Kim and I were very fortunate to be able to rent a lovely Victorian property called Crown East Cottage that overlooked the wood; and this enabled us to have lots of visitors who came for our guided walks and other events. The cottage was quite large and had 3 bedrooms, 2 reception rooms and a conservatory at the back and for the first few years it was adequate for our needs, but as our business grew we realized that we needed to find larger premises. We were now having groups of up to 30 people at times and in inclement weather we had nowhere to put them!

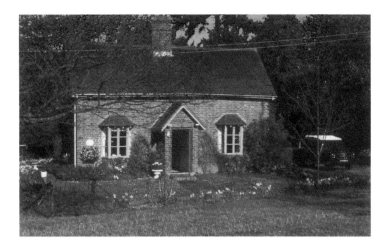

I was now working full time managing the woodland, Kim and I both enjoyed working with people and this made up for the fact that we made little or no profit but there were compensations because the location of the wood and view from cottage of the 'Malvern Hills' was amazing. It was also very rewarding to see the happy faces of our visitors and the results of our hard work as we reclaimed the neglected woodland back to its former glory.

View from the cottage

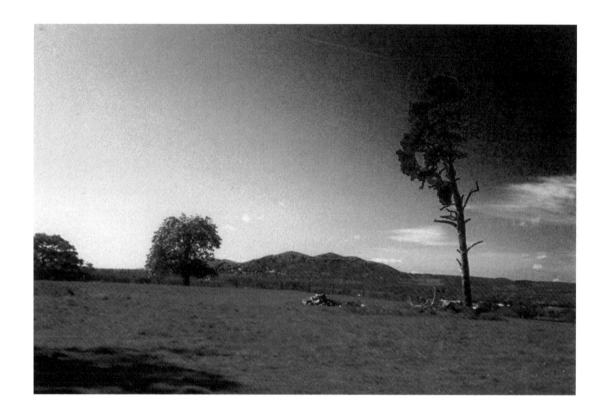

CROWN EAST HERITAGE WOODLAND

Winter   Bluebells in the Spring

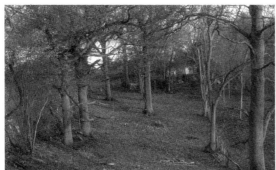 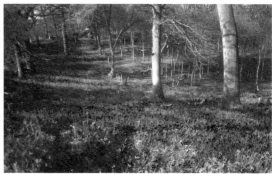

For a year we had been trying to secure planning approval for a woodland visitor centre, the building would enable us to earn more money in inclement weather by offering indoor facilities such as a lecture theatre and a class room for the schools and colleges that came, but the planners were having none of it. Eventually, after two failed applications, we opted for an inspector's inquiry but we lost our appeal and it was too much for us to bear. Kim and I had worked seven days a week for ten years trying desperately to earn a living while balancing the needs of the natural environment and we were very upset that the planners had been so short sighted; it was at this point that we had to sell the woodland because we had reached the end of the road with no way to accommodate our growing numbers of visitors and earn sufficient income.

MY FIRST REIKI TREATMENT

By now Kim and I were suffering from the effects of our failed planning applications and during this stressful period I developed Gout, a painful condition that was triggered by a combination of stress and a radical high protein diet that was fashionable at the time! I was prescribed powerful medication to keep the pain and symptoms under control but my condition got progressively worse over time and a friend of mine advised me to try a clinic in Worcester that offered alternative medicine such as acupuncture, reflexology, homeopathy and Reiki. I had tried acupuncture and reflexology some years earlier while I was waiting for my surgery and had found them both very effective. I had never heard of Reiki though, but was assured that it was very good for pain relief and was also a very balancing treatment. The following day I went to discuss my condition with the Reiki Master at the clinic who agreed that a treatment might help so I booked a session for the following day. I woke up the next morning in excruciating pain and my foot was hot, red and swollen, these were the classic symptoms of Gout so I decided that this would be a good opportunity to test the effectiveness of the treatment.

An hour later Kim drove me to the clinic, I hobbled in feeling rather awkward because I was carrying my shoe and sock in my hand because my foot was so painful and swollen that I couldn't put them on. I was led into a treatment room at the back of the clinic where the Reiki Master asked me to complete a medical questionnaire; I was also asked a few questions and was then told to lie on the Reiki table. At this point I didn't really know what a Reiki treatment was, but I was so desperate that I was willing to try anything to ease the pain.

I was afraid that the practitioner would hurt my painful foot so I asked her not to touch it under any circumstances; she smiled and assured me that there was no need for her to touch my foot at all! I was a little confused by her remarks and it made me think, how was she going to help me if she was not going to touch my foot?

So, there I was, lying on the table not knowing whether to laugh or cry as she explained what she was going to do. She mentioned 'Chakras' and energy meridians, 'Life force energy' and I felt very confused so I just nodded and pretended to understand what she was saying and presumed that *she* knew what she was talking about!

After a while, she placed her hands on my head and that was when I first noticed how hot her hands were and within minutes I fell fast asleep! Thirty minutes later she woke me and asked me to turn over on to my stomach then she placed her hands on my shoulders and I promptly fell asleep again!

In what seemed like the blink of an eye, she woke me again and told me that the treatment was over and I was given a glass of water to drink and asked to pay at the reception desk on the way out.

Kim was waiting for me outside and she gave me a peculiar look as I got into the car and then she asked me, "How did you get your shoe and sock on"? It was only then that I realized that I had no pain in my foot! The strange thing was that I had put my shoes and socks on and had not even noticed or thought about Gout but I admit that I felt a little 'spaced out,' but was so relaxed that I didn't care!

As soon as we arrived home I took my shoe and sock off because I wanted to take a look at my foot and I had a surprise! There was no sign of redness, swelling or pain and this really excited me because in the past when I had a reoccurrence of the symptoms, it took 4 or 5 days for them to subside and this treatment had done it in an hour!

Over the next few days I did some research about Reiki on the internet, some of the claims that were being made sounded far too good to be true but on the other hand, I had experienced something that I couldn't explain and *my* results spoke for themselves.

My Reiki treatment had taken away the pain and symptoms in a short period of time and that was something that powerful drugs had not been unable to do and I was impressed! The following day Kim told Linda, one of her colleagues at work what had happened to me, she didn't seem at all surprised to hear about my experience; in fact, it was then that she told Kim that she was a Reiki Master herself, what a coincidence! Linda mentioned that she was running a Reiki 1 course the following month and I was so intrigued that I booked myself on the course.

MY INITIATION INTO REIKI 1

It was the day of my course and I drove towards the wilds of the 'Clee Hills' in Shropshire in anticipation of what was to come. When I arrived Linda introduced me to the other students and I felt comfortable and relaxed as we chatted to each other.

Linda had given me some pre-course literature to read a few days before, but in all honesty I didn't really understand the terminology of what I was reading, but I guess that this was as good a reason as any to do the course, to find out!

The course lasted a day and what a day it turned out to be! Linda was a lovely woman; she had an air about her that was very calming, we were all given a Reiki manual and Linda periodically talked us through some of the contents before starting the 'attunements.'

Now, I want you to try to picture this. There were 5 straight backed chairs arranged side by side and we were asked to pick a chair and sit on it. I was third in line and Linda slowly and methodically did the attunements on each of the students, then she stood behind me. She placed her hands on my shoulders first and the heat from her hands seemed to penetrate deep into my body. Then she moved her hands onto the top of my head and a minute or two later she blew on the top of my head then something strange and wonderful happened. My eyes were closed at this point, but I saw a vivid indigo blue sky that was full of twinkling stars and one star in particular that was brighter than the rest caught my eye and I couldn't take my eyes off it. As I sat there transfixed, the star seemed to be getting bigger and closer to me and eventually I could see that it wasn't a star at all, it was a Unicorn and it was galloping straight towards me! The next thing that I felt was a judder as something entered the top of my head and I felt a surge of energy curse through my body and into my hands which made them feel very hot.

Linda then moved on to the next student and a short time later the first part of the attunement was over. We were then offered a glass of water and asked in turn if we had felt anything from the process. The first woman started to describe what she had experienced and I waited patiently for her to tell us about the Unicorn, but she didn't mention one! She did mention some unusual sensations that she had felt and so did the woman sitting next to her and now it was my turn!

I took a deep breath then explained what I had seen and what had happened to my hands! Everyone except Linda was astonished at what came out of my mouth, I was really none the wiser but I was enjoying every minute of my initiation into Reiki 1 because it was a new and exciting experience.

Finally, Linda completed the other attunements and it was now time to go. The day had gone so quickly and it was hard to describe what I was feeling because it was a strange mixture of calmness, heat in my hands and something else that I couldn't quite put my finger on. By now it was dark and very foggy outside, it had taken me an hour and a half to drive from Worcester in the morning and I didn't like the idea of driving home in thick fog but before I knew it, I was pulling onto my driveway at Crown East and to this day, I don't remember that journey home through the fog!

The next few weeks were a revelation for me with my 'new pair of Reiki hands.' Every time I did a treatment I experienced some new and unusual sensations in my hands. Sometimes they would heat up and on other occasions they felt like they were vibrating or were icy cold! The problem was that the more sensations I felt, the more confused I became and I wondered whether I had overlooked something during my training.

My Reiki 2 attunement

Three months later Linda contacted me to inform me that she was running a Reiki 2 class and asked me if I would be interested, *would I be interested?* I couldn't wait to do my second level because I was intrigued to find out what this higher level of Reiki felt like and I jumped at the chance.

Unlike the first course, the attunement for Reiki 2 was much shorter and was over in no time at all, although it still took another 7 hours to complete the course, we had to learn how to draw the 3 Reiki symbols and were told and shown how, and when to use them.

Over a period of time these symbols were to have a powerful effect on me and my clients. Linda had shown us how to send Reiki to people; the technique was called distant healing and at the time I thought that I would never be able to do this, but gradually I had proof from my clients that it worked and I began to use the symbols for most of my treatments. By now I was treating anyone and everyone that I could get my hands on, but I still wanted more people to practice on! I was learning fast now and I wanted to 'fix' everyone and then it dawned on me, I was not fixing *anyone*, my clients were fixing themselves. I will explain later!

My Reiki Master – Teacher attunement

As I discovered more about how Reiki worked I was fascinated with the idea that one day I might 'become' a Reiki Master, then out of the blue Linda offered to do the A.R.T., advanced Reiki training and Master – Teacher attunement for me. After the attunement I was in awe at the power that flowed from my hands and then the reality dawned on me that all I really needed to do was place my hands on, or near someone and Reiki would flow to where it was needed. I must admit that at the time I didn't fully understand the intricacies of how this was possible but I kept seeing positive results time and time again from the treatments and learnt to just accept that this was the way it was.

Some Usui, Tibetan Reiki, and Non-traditional symbols

Here are some of the Reiki symbols that maybe used during an attunement.

The symbols are drawn onto various parts of the body during the attunement process. These areas include the palms of the hands, Crown and the third eye.

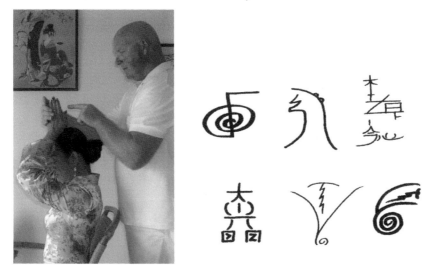

Reiki symbols being drawn down the spine, over the hands and into the third eye during an attunement.

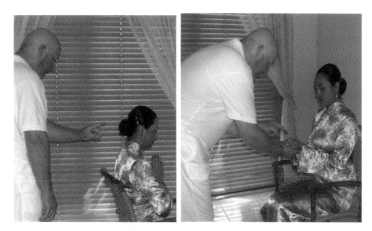

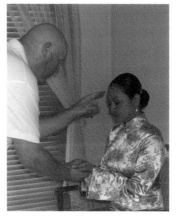

The symbols are drawn over the energy centres and are visualized, 'tapped' and 'blown' into the chakras and are then absorbed into the students energy field.

Chapter 6

AS ONE DOOR CLOSES...

After we lost our planning appeal we had to sell the woodland and we decided to move out of our cottage. It was a bitter pill to swallow because we had little or no choice and Kim and I agreed that we would have an open weekend at the cottage to have a house contents sale. Everything we owned had to go, including our Chickens and ducks and it was a very sad day for everyone, especially our loyal customers who had become our friends over the years.

Crown East Cottage

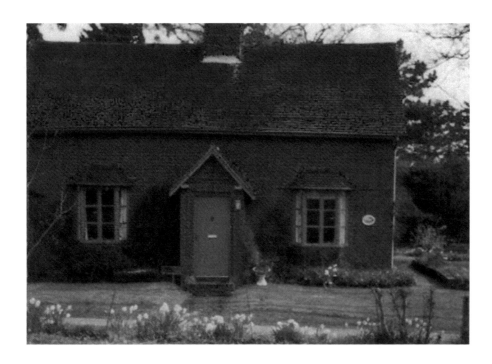

Our Chickens   and   Ducklings

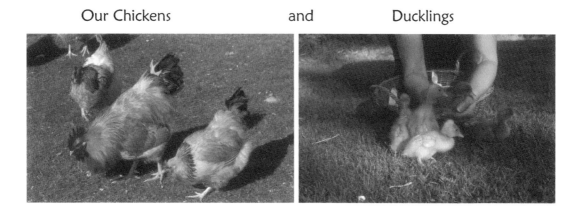

The last day dawned and as we walked through the bluebells for the last time the enormity of what had happened to us sank in. It had been an amazing voyage of discovery, we had worked with nature for 10 wonderful years and now it was time to move on.

We were now both in need of a break and a few weeks later we boarded a plane for a holiday to Cyprus. Almost everyone on the island spoke English and with no language barriers for us to overcome the thought crossed our minds that Cyprus might be a good place for us to re-locate to. And a short time later our minds were made up.

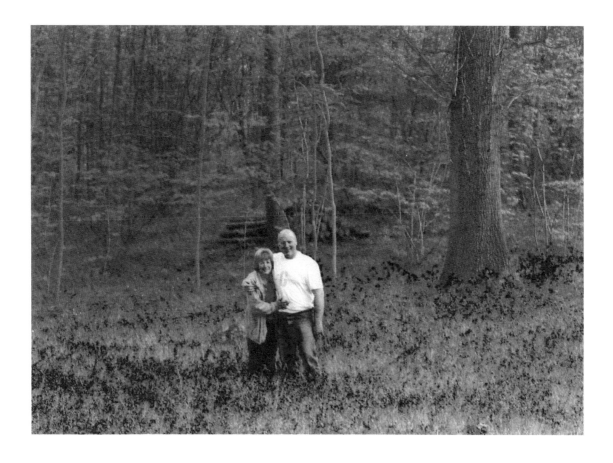

A New Life in Cyprus

We left England and arrived in Cyprus in early June to begin our new adventure. It was my intention to look for work in nature conservation because there were numerous nature reserves on the island. I sent my C.V. with a covering letter to the Cyprus forestry service to see if they had any vacancies but a month later; I received a curt one-line reply informing me that there was no work for me in nature conservation on the island! This came as a shock to me because now I had to think of another means of earning a living.

The journey of a lifetime begins.

It was now time to put plan B into operation and I decided that I would practice Reiki! I started by visiting 5 star Hotels in Paphos where I lived to see if any of the Spa managers would be interested in having Reiki in their Spa menus. At first I was not taken seriously because no one had heard of 'Reiki' but I was not going to give up yet because I had decided that this was to become my new career and I eventually found part-time work in four hotels. Treatments were slow in coming at first; and I really had to convince the guests about the benefits of having a Reiki treatment and then it dawned on me, hardly any of the guests knew what Reiki was! I decided to offer Reiki taster sessions for the hotel guests as I thought that this might encourage them to come along and sample some Reiki for themselves.

I had never done anything like this before, but I knew that previously some of my clients had felt the flow of Reiki from my hands and I decided that this would be the starting point for the sessions.

It was 10am in the morning and I had my first group of people standing in front of me, I briefly explained the origins of Reiki, where it was discovered and what Reiki was etc. then i asked one of the guests to hold out his hands. I held my hands about 6 inches beneath his and tentatively waited to see what happened. I instantly felt a flow of Reiki from my hands as the energy was *taken* by the guest and he made a comment that his hands were 'tingling' as if a mild electrical current was passing over and through his fingers and said how strange it felt! "Yes" I thought, thank god that he felt something!

The list of sensations that this first group of people experienced was impressive, some individuals felt tingling sensations, while others felt heat, cold or a magnetic pull or push from my hands and they were really impressed and intrigued by what they felt.

Every time I did a taster session I learnt something new about Reiki and this was part of my on-going Reiki apprenticeship.

The sessions were my key to success because within a short period of time guests were recommending Reiki to other people that they had met in the Hotel. This was all the encouragement that I needed and it spurred me on to think of other ways of introducing Reiki to those who had never heard of it.

I approached a couple of editors of ex-pat magazines to see if they would give me some editorial in exchange for Reiki treatments for their staff, "This was fine" I was told, but I would need to advertise with them first to have some 'free' editorial! I decided to take them up on their offer and every month I wrote articles about Reiki and advertised the courses that I was teaching at week-ends.

This was the beginning of a steep learning curve for me because Reiki was teaching me things that I had not read in books. For the most part, I didn't know what to expect and it was just as well because some of the things that I saw were bizarre to say the least!

Chapter 7

CASE STUDY 1: CATCHING THE FLU CAN TEACH YOU SOMETHING!

I was now using Reiki symbols that I had been attuned to on a daily basis. The symbols sometimes made a huge difference to the outcome of the treatments, but I was still learning how best to use them and on a number of occasions the effects that I got when I used them took me completely by surprise!

I remember one treatment very well; I had just treated a young woman called Michelle. She really enjoyed the session, and by the end of her treatment felt relaxed, calm and energized all at the same time. She asked me if I had treated anyone with the flu before because her boyfriend had been laid up in bed in the Hotel for the past 2 days and felt really awful.

I had not had the opportunity to treat anyone with the flu before but said that if she could persuade him to come to the Spa, it might be worth trying a treatment.

Several minutes later I was called to the Spa reception and standing there looking awful was Michelle's boyfriend Andy. His face was flushed, he was shivering and sweating profusely and it was at this point that I felt really guilty about getting him out of his sick bed. I hoped that the treatment would help to alleviate some of his symptoms and I thanked him for taking the time to come to the spa.

I then asked him how he felt and he said "like death," so as soon as I had booked him in with the reception, I took him to my room.

Because he looked so ill, I decided to use six Reiki symbols that I was attuned too, so I drew them over his energy centres as I came to them. Within a short period of time; about fifteen minutes, I began to see an improvement in his condition.

The first thing I noticed was that he had stopped sweating and when I placed my hands on his body, I could feel that his temperature had dropped and his face was not flushed anymore. And a few minutes later he fell fast asleep and I had to wake him to turn him over onto his stomach. He then fell asleep again. During the second half of the treatment he didn't move a muscle. He slept soundly and breathed easily, and this was in total contrast to how he had been earlier when he said that he felt congested.

With the treatment over, I gently woke him and sat him up. He had a long drink of water and when I asked him, said that he felt fine.

He then explained that he had not heard of Reiki before until Michelle had dragged him out of bed and he only agreed to have the treatment "to keep her happy."

As Andy got off the couch he gave me a *look*; this was a sign that 'something special' had happened, he thanked me for the treatment and made his way back to the hotel. The following day he and Michelle came back to the Spa to speak to me.

Andy looked really well and he had no signs of the 'flu' or any of the symptoms that he had exhibited the day before. He told me that as he walked back to the Hotel, he had felt no signs of the weakness and shakiness that he had come with earlier and when he got back to his room, Michelle couldn't believe her eyes because he looked so much better! Andy told her that he felt hungry which came as no surprise to Michelle because he hadn't eaten anything for two days, so he showered, got dressed and the both of them went for their first proper meal in two days.

At this point the Spa receptionist made a comment that "Andy looked amazing."

Andy and Michelle had come to thank me for the treatment, but this was a dual benefit for both of us because I had learnt a great deal from his treatment that day about the effectiveness of 'Life force energy.'

My new insight and sensory awareness

Reiki was giving me new experiences every day now and some of these were strange, bizarre and weird to say the least, and my clients started to utter these three words when they were trying to describe their treatments. It became clear to me that Reiki was slowly introducing me to some new ways of helping my clients.

There were days when I would 'mix and match' the Reiki symbols during the treatments to try to ascertain which ones were the right ones to use, sometimes I would draw a single symbol onto someone and the effect was instant and I knew that my intuition had guided me to choose the right symbol for this particular client. There were other occasions however when I wasn't so sure which ones to use, so I took no chances and used all six, there was no harm done because the clients' energy centres' could decide where the symbols were needed and would absorb them into their system if necessary.

Up to this point I had learnt some valuable lessons, I found that the clients brain was rarely instrumental in effecting the best outcome from the treatment, their chakras, or 'energy centres' on the other hand would always strive to bring about a positive result. I now know that the brain does not always control the chakra's function because the chakras work independently and only on rare occasions did I see an overriding effect from the brain and this invariably resulted in a negative outcome for the client.

There was something else that intrigued me, sometimes when I drew a symbol over a chakra the client appeared to response in a negative way and would sometimes cry, but by the end of the treatment would say that they felt so much better. It then became obvious that the tears that the client had cried were not the normal tears that we would cry ourselves. The Reiki energy had released so much more than tear drops; it had gone to the core of the problem to release their deep seated emotions.

You may have heard the expression, "Have a good cry it will make you feel better," well, I knew that this was rarely the case because it was possible for someone to cry for a week and still feel dreadful. Tears are an indication of the pain that we are suffering and in the case of a Reiki treatment; if you cry during a treatment you can be assured that you are well on the road to recovery.

Of course, all tears are not necessarily caused by our negative emotions because we cry for many reasons, especially when we are happy and filled with joy.

CASE STUDY 2: JOAN'S PERSONAL LOSS

Joan was on holiday, she had decided to book herself a Reiki treatment because she had not experienced one before. When I was first introduced to her, I first sensed that there was a gentle energy radiating from her, but there was also sadness.

She looked to be in her mid-fifties, was immaculately dressed and had shiny black hair and a lovely smile.

For some time now I had used essential oils and candles during my treatments and on this occasion I decided to add some Lavender oil to my oil burner. Joan made a comment that she loved the smell of lavender and she had recently purchased a Lavender pillow for her bed to help her sleep.

As I started her treatment I became aware of a sense of calmness around me, but it also felt as though I was in a vacuum and insulated from the out-side world.

I also had the feeling that *something* unusual was about to happen, but I didn't know what that *something* was and then within a minute or two Joan fell fast asleep. Several minutes had passed since I started the treatment then I noticed something by her feet that caught my eye. I could see what I thought were a number of small round globes. There were some holes cut out from the sides of my oil burner that would have cast a distinctive shadow on the wall by her feet but none of these were circular in shape so I discounted these.

My eyes were now transfixed on the globes because they were moving randomly around in circles and then they rose up into the air and appeared to go straight through the ceiling! What on earth were they and where had they come from?

For a minute or two I looked around the room, everything looked the same, my oil burner and the light from the corridor; there were no other light sources anywhere and I was completely baffled!

At this point, my mind came back to the job in hand, and I felt a little guilty because I didn't normally get distracted during a treatment, but this was an exception.

Now as I looked at Joan's face she started to smile, she sounded fast asleep, her breathing was deep and her eyes were closed so I presumed that she must be dreaming. I carried on with the treatment and when I finished I asked her how she was feeling. She started to cry very gently and smile at the same time and I presumed that this meant that she felt happy. I had seen tears like this before and knew that her tears were from something that had left her feeling deeply moved, and in a comforting way. I offered her a tissue to wipe her eyes then she told me about her son Paul.

He had been unhappy for a long period of time and this had left him feeling very depressed and tragically, he took his own life, he was just 20 years old.

Joan had struggled to come to terms with his death, she felt guilty, after all, she was his mother and she was supposed to take care of him! She should have seen the danger signs and prevented his suicide, this was how she felt.

I explained to her that the closer you are to someone, the more difficult it is to see the obvious, after all, who expects their child to commit suicide?

It had been 2 years since Paul's death and it had left her feeling empty inside, that is, until today. Now she wanted to tell me about her wonderful treatment.

She said that in an instant, the warmth from my hands had relaxed her, she then felt herself drift off to sleep and found herself in a wonderful place. She could still hear the music from my CD and she felt that she was not asleep or awake but somewhere in between. She saw herself walking in a wonderful garden, she could smell the perfume from the summer flowers, feel the warm sun on her face and the breeze in her hair and she could also see the silhouette of a man standing in the distance. As she walked towards him she was surprised to see that it was her son Paul. He put his arms around her and she could feel the strength of his arms holding her tight and at this point she knew that somehow this was not a dream.

Tears were running down her cheeks, but she was still smiling as she told me that Paul apologized to her for all the pain he had caused her. He had never meant to hurt her, his life was just too much to bear and it was because of this that he had to stop the pain. He said that he was happy now and it was not her fault that he had taken his life.

Joan was now calm and elated because this was the first time since Paul had died that she felt at peace. She knew that what she had just experienced was real, she was definitely not asleep and the experience had left her feeling wonderful, she then gave me a big hug and thanked me for the treatment. By now I was feeling quite emotional myself, but in a way that was rewarding.

Some months later I was watching a program about the paranormal and a few minutes into the documentary it showed an infra-red camera picking up something in a room that was in total darkness and I instantly recognized that these were the globes that I had seen in the room during Joan's treatment!

The commentary said that these were called 'Orbs,' and that orbs are associated with haunted buildings and paranormal activity and they were usually a pre-curser for a spirit to manifest itself. Everything made sense now because when I had first seen the orbs, Joan had been 'talking' to her dead son's energy, how amazing was that!

I have seen orbs on several occasions since treating Joan and it has always been a wonderful experience for me and my clients. A spiritual connection takes place during these treatments that makes them very special; it's a link to the spirit world that takes place when it is needed.

CASE STUDY 3: IT'S A DOG'S LIFE

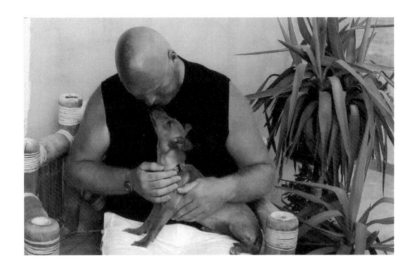

Ann loved animals and she had recently 'acquired' a little dog from the rescue centre. She was determined to make sure that her dog would have a healthy and happy life and to this end asked the vet to immunize him before she brought him home. Unfortunately, 'Oscar' had been off his food since his inoculations and had not drunk any water for the past two days. Ann was worried, her little dog looked sick. His nose was dry and his coat had lost its sheen.

I had been invited to Ann's house for a BBQ and as soon as I saw her dog I knew that something was wrong. 'Oscar' was lying on the grass, he looked very sorry for himself and I asked Ann what was wrong with him. She told me about his 'Jabs' and the fact that he was off his food and asked me if I would give him some Reiki. I said that Reiki was an excellent way to treat sick animals as they usually responded to it very well, and at that, I picked up the dog and gently sat him on my lap. Almost straight away, I felt him taking some Reiki and my hands began to tingling and get really hot. After a few minutes, he jumped down from my lap and ran off; Ann and I were both amazed! Then a couple of minutes later he returned and we noticed his wet nose, then he started to play with his toys and he ran about as if there was nothing wrong with him! I asked Ann to give him something to eat so she put some chicken in his dish and as soon as he saw it, he polished it off in a flash; Ann commented that she had tried to feed him earlier and he had turned his nose up at the food and walked away! I then poured some water into his bowl and he lapped up every last drop so I filled his dish again and he drank a little more before running off to play again and now he was showing off to everyone and having a wonderful time of it all.

Whatever had been wrong with him had completely disappeared within a few minutes of having the treatment and Ann was delighted. She couldn't believe what her eyes had seen and I must admit it was quite remarkable to see such an improvement in such a short period of time.

Treating animals is very rewarding for me because I don't have to convince them about Reiki, they either take it, or they don't, and when they have taken enough they usually get up and walk away.

CASE STUDY 4: A SHOCK TO HIS SYSTEM!

Jeff had decided that he just had to get away, he needed a holiday and the chance to recover from the stress that he was suffering from, he had been working long hours, and felt as if he was sinking fast, his life seemed to be out of control and no matter how hard he worked, it made no difference to his workload. He had discussed his problems with one of my colleagues while he was having a massage and she recommended that he should try a Reiki treatment. He had never heard of Reiki before and was a little apprehensive about trying something new so I explained that a Reiki treatment can sometimes help to balance the emotions and if he was feeling stressed, a Reiki treatment might be just what he needed. It was obvious that he had a nervous disposition and he looked very vulnerable and I could 'feel' his emotional pain.

At this point Jeff he asked me if it was possible for him to have a 30 minute treatment, I suspected that this was because he wanted to get it over and done with as soon as possible! I advised him to have a full treatment because a short treatment may help to reduce his stress levels, but if he were to have a full treatment, there were other options that I could use to target the emotions that were having an adverse effect on his life. After thinking about it for a while he decided that a full treatment seemed a better option, he then completed his medical questionnaire and lay on the table for his treatment.

From the outset, this was to be an unusual treatment and after few seconds he nearly jumped off the couch and this took me completely by surprise. I had felt him twitch violently just before he jumped, but it was as if he had received an electric shock and three or four minutes later it happened again, only this time I sensed something 'building.' It felt like there was a Volcano about to erupt beneath my hands, but the sensations that I felt were not in my hands, they were felt inwardly by my intuition. I knew instinctively that his stress was being held in his sacral chakra, this area of the body is also called the tanden or hara. It is situated approximately 3 inches below the navel and is an area that we sometimes store our emotional tension in, and this was certainly the case with Jeff.

As I placed my hands over his tanden he began to sob uncontrollably, I kept my hands there for about 6 minutes until the sensations in my hands subsided and it was at this point that he fell asleep. The second half of the treatment was uneventful because he slept like a baby all the way through it.

It was now time for me to ask some questions so I asked Jeff to describe his treatment to me. He now looked more relaxed and said that although he had 'jumped' so much during the first half of the treatment, this was not because of any painful sensations; it was just how his body reacted to the energy. In fact, he had felt something brewing up inside him before it was released and he said that it was quite a pleasant sensation! "Quite a pleasant sensation"! *His* reaction had nearly given me a heart attack!

This just goes to show that it is prudent to ask what a client is feeling during or after the treatment because I had made the assumption from what I had seen that his sensations were far from pleasant. This was one of the defining treatments that I will never forget and now if something unusual happens during a treatment, I ask what the recipient is feeling. I had learnt another valuable lesson.

CASE STUDY 5: A DEPRESSED ARTIST

Talking or even thinking about depression makes me feel 'low,' and I must admit that I have never suffered from depression myself, but I have met and treated many clients who were suffering from this debilitating illness. I am no expert on the subject but I know that there can be numerous causes of the illness such as hormone imbalance and physical or emotional trauma. The latter may cause post-traumatic stress disorder and may well be responsible for bringing about a depressed state and these are just a few examples! It would be wrong of me to generalize, so I will only discuss the beneficial effects of Reiki treatments on clients that I have treated personally.

James was a talented artist, his paintings were amazing but for the past three years he had suffered from chronic depression and his life had become meaningless and his depression was having a devastating effect on his life. He had lost the will to paint, didn't want to get out of bed in the morning and found life in general very difficult.

His wife Mary had recently read an article in a magazine that I wrote about Reiki and depression and thought that James should try a treatment.

When she phoned to ask me if a Reiki treatment might help, I said I felt sure that her husband would get some benefit from the treatment so she booked him in for a treatment the following day.

When he arrived, it was easy to see why his wife was worried about him; I could see the devastating effects of the depression written all over his face.

Once he had completed the medical questionnaire I got to work on him straight away and within minutes he fell fast asleep and apart from that, nothing of any significance happened during the treatment that I could see or feel.

An hour later, I woke him up and gave him a glass of water while I completed my post treatment notes and it was while I was doing this that I noticed a difference in him.

Firstly, he looked different; he was far more relaxed now than he had been an hour earlier and there was something else that was different about him, he was smiling.

Whatever had happened to him during the treatment had left the room feeling 'Happy' and this was another indication that there was a change in his condition.

James was somewhat of an introvert; perhaps this was because he was shy, or just didn't feel the need to say anything to me but after the treatment I felt that somehow he had turned a corner with his health.

I asked him to call me a few days later just to let me know how he was feeling, he agreed, then he went on his way.

The following afternoon, Mary phoned me, she sounded very excited and told me that James was "himself again." She said that this morning he got out of bed early, made her a cup of tea and acted completely differently and appeared to be happy and was smiling which had not happened for a very long time!

She decided that he ought to have another treatment so I booked him in for another a few days later and when he arrived for his treatment, I couldn't believe the difference in him. He looked great and I could feel the energy radiating from him and it was hard to believe that this was the same man that I had treated only a week earlier.

His second treatment, was similar to the first one, the only difference was that this time when he fell asleep the Reiki energy seemed to regulate his breathing because it got deeper and more relaxed as the treatment progressed.

When I woke him up at the end of the treatment, he commented that he had "been on an amazing journey," he hadn't recognized where he was, but he had seen a beautiful garden full of flowers, birds and animals. It was so real that he felt sure he was there and not just dreaming because he had felt my hands on his body when I moved them from one position to another. He said that now, he felt so calm and relaxed and had never felt like this in his entire life before. I believed him because I could feel an air of his calmness in the room; I had also heard something similar from other clients when they described their treatments.

He was indeed a changed man, firstly he was now talking to me as if he had known me for a lifetime and this was certainly very different than how he had been previously and I could hardly get a word in!

The results of this second treatment were revealed to me a few days later when Mary called me. She told me about the amazing transformation that had taken place with her husband and half way through a sentence, she broke down and cried. Between the tears, she thanked me for "returning her husband to her" and for lifting him out of the black depression that he had endured for so long. I said that I was the one who should be thanking him, because he had given me the opportunity to learn from the experience, and I could relate to his illness because I had felt his emotional state. James had made a rapid recovery from his illness because *he had taken his medication*. That medication was the Reiki energy that was available to him during the treatment and the energy was not given to him by me, because it was not mine to give, he had healed himself.

CASE STUDY 6: NO LIFE AT ALL

Maria came to me in desperation, she was a young woman in her early twenties but the effects of her illness made her look much older than her years. She was suffering from depression and had been taking anti-depressants for over a year, the medication helped her get through the day but left her feeling 'spaced out and distant' and only masked the cause of her condition. She had also read one of my articles about depression and thought a Reiki treatment might help her.

From the outset, I decided to use the mental/emotional and the distant healing symbol in her session because these symbols can be used at any time and can be of huge benefit when looking for the cause of an illness or imbalance.

During my Master/Teacher training I was attuned to 6 Reiki symbols, some of these symbols enable the practitioner to work on blockages that may be lodged in the clients' subconscious mind. The distant healing symbol for example can be used to send Reiki backwards or forwards in time, a technique called 'Distant Healing.' I thought that if I used this symbol in combination with the others, they may release some, if not all of the blockages that may have caused Maria's depression. I had seen some good results from this method of using Reiki on other occasions and felt confident that she would get some benefits from the treatment. I also mentioned to her that sometimes this technique can be emotionally painful, but in my opinion it was worth trying and she agreed to go ahead. I decided to spend a larger proportion of the treatment working on Maria's Brow chakra and I would draw the mental - emotional symbol over her 'Third Eye' and if the cause of her depression was an emotional trauma then Reiki would hopefully release it.

I started by drawing the symbols over the chakra, her eyes were closed but the effect of drawing them was instantaneous because Maria began to smile. The symbols had expanded her consciousness and triggered a reaction and I wondered what she was feeling, I was sure it was something pleasant so I continued with the treatment and placed my hand over her brow. She then started to laugh and her laughter was so contagious that I started to laugh too and for the next few minutes we couldn't help ourselves and it felt great!

After a few minutes I composed myself and asked Maria how she felt, although I could see the effect of the treatment on her face. Her eyes were sparkling and she had a grin on her face from ear to ear, this was in total contrast to how she had been before because her eyes had appeared 'lifeless and empty.'

It was now time for her to tell me how she felt, she said that something had touched her deep inside but that it was difficult to explain exactly what that something was, she did however say that she felt amazing. I had seen treatments like this before and I knew what she was feeling, it is the one thing that everyone needs in their lives, *Joy*!

I asked her if there was anything she could compare her feelings with; she paused for a moment, blushed and said that it felt like 'being in love.' She then asked me if everyone felt this good after a Reiki treatment and I explained that everyone has different needs and it is those needs that determine the outcome of the treatment.

Here is an example of how Reiki can work for your best interests.

A client may *think* that they know what their needs are but the reality is sometimes quite different. Our chakras know what is best for us and it is a combination of this 'chakra knowledge' and the Reiki symbols that create the ideal conditions to heal and balance us. The chakras are able to work independently without the help of our brain if we let them and this will create a balance, but the Chakras can also be adversely affected by our negative thoughts because these thoughts can deplete our 'Life-force energy.'

Several weeks later I bumped into Maria in the supermarket, she looked amazing and I could feel the 'life-force energy' emanating from her. I asked her how she had been since the treatment and her reply was just what I wanted to hear. She said that from the moment I started the treatment, she had not felt depressed at all and said that Reiki was amazing. She had never felt better in her life and as she walked way, I couldn't help thinking what a difference one treatment can make to a persons' life.

COMBINING EMOTIONAL AND DISTANT HEALING DURING A TREATMENT

Distant healing can be used when the practitioner is aware of an emotional issue or imbalance. This *awareness* may be because you were informed by a client that there are some emotional issues that need resolving, or the practitioner may just *feel* or *sense* the emotional condition of a client, in either case, permission should be sought before commencing the treatment. The reason for this is that sometimes a treatment can be painful for the client because longstanding emotional issues may be brought to the surface for them to deal with before the healing can take place.

These emotional issue may be from the past, perhaps, from many years ago. The length of time that you have had the issue is not a problem for the practitioner, but it can be for the client because it may have had a long lasting negative effect on their health and wellbeing. When using distant healing, it is possible to send Reiki back in time to deal with these emotional issues and if the practitioner is aware that there is an emotional blockage, he or she can use the emotional symbol to address the situation.

The Distant healing symbol (that I use)   The Emotional symbol

I use these symbols on a daily basis and have learnt to trust them because they work!

CASE STUDY 7: A REIKI SEMINAR

I was giving a Reiki seminar to a group of people and noticed that one of them had his wrist in a plaster cast, I asked him what he had done to it and he said that he had fallen over and broken it in two places. I asked him if it was still painful and he replied that it was, and that his fingers were still swollen.

I thought that this might be a good opportunity to see if Reiki could ease the pain, so I offered to give him a few minutes of Reiki to put Reiki to the test. I decided that I would not touch the plaster cast; I would merely hold my hands a couple of inches away from the plaster to see if anything happened.

Adam had not heard of Reiki before, and didn't really understand the concept of healing energy, so was a little sceptic about it, but that didn't stop him wanting to try it, so I started the treatment by drawing some Reiki symbols over the cast. I didn't touch it at this point, but Adam looked puzzled because as I drew the symbols, he felt a strange sensation under the cast!

Before I started, his wrist and fingers were aching and after I drew the symbols over the cast, the ache changed to a 'tingle' and now while I was holding my hands next to the plaster the 'tingling' sensations became stronger. By this time, *my* hands were getting very hot and they were also 'tingling.' I held my hands there next to the cast until the sensations in my hands subsided and then asked Adam to tell me what his wrist felt like.

He gave me *that* look, the one that says 'I don't believe this.' He explained that immediately I had placed my hands next to the plaster cast, the pain had subsided and been replaced by a 'tingling' sensation, it felt like his wrist had 'gone to sleep,' then, the 'tingling faded away and the pain had gone with it!

The other guests at the seminar asked me how this was possible and said "How is it that there are not more Reiki healers?" "That's a good question" I said, and one that I find difficult to explain because I have seen some amazing treatments, but I am still only a novice in terms of understanding the full potential that Reiki has to offer us.

My personal experiences are part of my apprenticeship and Reiki is continually up-grading my personal abilities. For me, treatments equal power, not power over my clients, but power that is available for them to take when it is required. One thing I cannot stress enough is that to empower yourself as a practitioner or Master, you have to do as many Reiki treatments as you can, this enables you to strengthen and build the 'life force energy that flows through you as a channel for others and the more treatments you do, the stronger a channel you become.

CASE STUDY 8: WAS THIS A CASE OF CHANCE OR FATE?

This treatment changed my opinion about what is 'meant to be,' you can call this fate, destiny or whatever you like but I know that some things are definitely meant to be.

I was sitting in the Spa reception area, when a couple came in and sat down opposite me. Peter spoke to me and asked about massage, he asked me if I was busy at this time of the year. I must add at this juncture that I have broad shoulders, a bald head and a huge pair of hands, so it was easy to see why he had made the presumption that I was a masseur. I said that I was a Reiki Master and then his wife Sarah said that she had heard of Reiki and that some of her friends had tried it. Peter was curious and asked me lots of questions, but unfortunately each time I answered a question, it led to another, this went on for a while and then he asked if I had time to give him a treatment today. Fortunately I had just enough time for one more treatment and without further delay I asked him to complete the Spa medical questionnaire and took him to my room.

It was at this point that he told me that he and his wife *usually* came into the Spa via another door, but on this occasion they had decided to come through the *other door* and this was the reason that they saw me sitting there.

Peter had a face that seemed very familiar to me and I asked him if we had met before, he said that he had not seen me before although he had been to Cyprus on several occasions, and said that maybe I had just seen him around.

I placed my hands on Peters head to start the treatment, then he interrupted me to ask a question. He asked me why he was having a problem keeping his arms on the couch, because since I put my hands on his head his arms seemed to want to lift up!

I replied that it was best to relax, and let his body do whatever it wanted to do, and not to 'fight it,' he thanked me then I felt his tension slip away as he relaxed into the treatment.

I resumed the hand position on his head and instantly his arms began to rise, then his legs and then his head and I thought, 'this was going to be one of *those* amazing treatments.' As the treatment progressed, Peter said that in all of his fifty years, nothing that he had ever experienced in his life could compare with this!

And with almost every placement of my hands, he had other remarkable experiences. Sometimes he would 'see' something although his eyes were closed, then I would move my hands and place them on the next energy centre and he would have a different sensation and on one occasion, his body arched into a 'v' shape and he had no control over what was happening.

I have to say that Peters' treatment was not unique, as I had witnessed a few like his in the last few years but never the less, they were all remarkable in one way or another.

When the treatment was over he asked me a question, "Did you hypnotize me?" he said, I said "Definitely not," I only practice and teach Reiki not Hypnotherapy!

Then I asked him why he thought I had hypnotized him and he said that he couldn't work it out, or believe what he had just seen and felt, and who would blame him!

I could tell that there was some doubt in Peters mind about being hypnotized, so I offered to prove to him in another way that I was genuine so I offered to *send* him some Reiki.

I could do this by arranging a time that was suitable for him, and then send him some 'Distant Healing.' The thought crossed my mind that this might be too much for him to take in, or believe but I knew from past experience that he would have the same reaction to Distant Healing as he would have if he was lying on my table in the treatment room so we agreed that I would send him Reiki at 7:00pm the following evening.

The only thing I asked him to do was to be either sitting or lying down and I would then send him some Reiki and he would know once and for all if he had any reactions from it.

The following evening I sat down at home at 6:45pm and prepared to send Distant Healing to him. I knew without a shadow of a doubt that this would convince Peter because he would feel the same sensations that he had felt the day before and I was pleased that he had agreed to take part in the exercise. Note, I didn't call this an experiment because I had sent Distant Healing many times before and knew that it worked.

At exactly 7pm I started sending Reiki to him, I decided that the treatment would last about fifteen minutes and at 7.20pm my phone rang, it was Peter and he sounded ecstatic. He said that he had 'floated' up again, and this time his wife Sarah had watched in amazement and they were both astounded. He said that he was now convinced that this was not the result of me hypnotizing him and he trusted Sarah to tell him the truth, and she did.

Peter and Sarah have kept in touch since his treatment and as I mentioned earlier, I had felt a strong energetic link between us the first time that we met.

While I was writing this book, I thought long and hard about who would find it appealing because I thought this was vital to the success of the publication. Then I had some inspiration. I meet a lot of people who are searching for something, so in terms of numbers, this book will be of interest to anyone who is looking for that special something. And maybe some of *your* answers will be in this book, or lead you in another direction altogether that will reveal what you need to know. In either case I hope you find your own 'Enlightenment' by reading it.

I have another important reason for writing about my Reiki experiences. If you have ever been disappointed or disillusioned about someone you will know how awful this can make you feel but if you find a friend, that friendship may last a lifetime. This was how I felt when I first discovered Reiki some years ago, I felt like I had found a long lost friend.

Case study 9: Crohn's disease

I thought I knew how Reiki worked then I got blown away by an unusual treatment.

Wendy was looking for ways to relax; she had crohn's disease which is a chronic debilitating disease of the large and small intestines. She was in constant pain and suffered from diarrhoea, cramps and constantly felt exhausted. Her friend recommended that she try a Reiki treatment as she was aware that it could be used for pain control.

I asked Wendy to lie on the couch and proceeded to 'scan' her. This is a Japanese technique for sensing imbalances called Byosen Scanning.

I scanned her body, moving my hands over the energy centres, as I went from one to the other she started to exhibit signs of chronic pain; this was in response to the Reiki energy, as her body absorbed and took what it needed. This took her and me completely by surprise.

When the scan was completed I started the treatment and as I moved from one hand placement to another I felt her taking huge amounts of Reiki. This confirmed her need for the energy and it was also an indication of the severity of her illness.

Throughout the treatment Wendy felt pain building up inside her beneath my hands, culminating with a release of that pain. What she was feeling is called a Reiki cycle. If my hands are kept in place for any length of time, more of these cycles occur. When these cycles stop, it's an indication to move to the next hand position.

By the end of her treatment she had felt a considerable amount of pain but the result was that not only was she now pain free, she felt comfortable and relaxed.

This was the first time I had treated anyone with the disease, so I had no measure to use as a rule of thumb but Reiki had produced a good result by removing the pain.

Some months later I had a similar case and the second treatment was almost identical to the first, the client felt an increase in pain during the treatment and the pain had subsided by the end. Now when I treat someone who has the disease, I am not surprised by what happens and can inform the client that he or she may have an increase in pain during the treatment but may well have a reduction of the symptoms by the end.

Keeping up to date with Reiki developments is much easier now that we have the internet because some practitioners tell us about their experiences and this has to be the way forward.

There has been an influx of new Reiki web sites and some of these offer updates describing Mikao Usui's original techniques and hand positions. These techniques have shed new light on how Usui sensei taught Reiki in Japan and this also indicates that Reiki is still a developing therapy.

For a couple of years now I have felt guided by my intuition, sometimes I instinctively knew that I had to skip a hand placement and move my hands to somewhere else, and on other occasions I would use just one finger on a chakra instead of two hands. At the time, I thought I should just do what I felt, instead of repeating the basic hand positions for every treatment. What my intuition showed me was a revelation. On every occasion that I did something different it was always beneficial to my client. I deduce from this that Reiki had heightened my intuitive abilities to enable me to give my clients the best possible outcome from their treatments.

This heightened intuition may be a natural progression for anyone who is continually doing lots of treatments and this gave me an idea. Was this how Mikao Usui chose his hand positions, through intuition? There are numerous Reiki books that mention the hand positions that he used. Recently a book was published showing some Usui techniques that were very different from these basic hand positions. I purchased this book in January 2009 and when I opened it I was surprised to see that a number of the photographs showed some of the hand positions that I had been doing intuitively before the book was even published!

This confirmed to me that when we are ready to receive it, Reiki enables us to channel the energy in a more focused and beneficial way, by guided intuition.

CASE STUDY 10: NIGHTMARES FROM THE PAST!

I had started work in a new Spa and the manager thought that it would be a good idea if the reception staff and therapists experienced a Reiki treatment for themselves because this would enable them to explain to guests what a Reiki treatment was and this was vital if Reiki was to be recommended to Spa guests.

The Spa was new and had only just been built and the manager decided to start with the reception staff. Jacky, the head receptionist told me that she had a friend who was a Reiki practitioner but she had not actually tried a treatment herself, although she had heard many stories about how wonderful Reiki therapy was.

I decided to give Jacky just a little information about the treatment and asked her not to discuss her treatment with anyone until I had treated everyone, this would help them to evaluate their experiences individually and not be influenced by each other's comments.

As I started her treatment, I felt the energy pulse through my hands, it was extremely powerful and after several minutes she began to cry very gently. Tears were trickling down her cheeks and I sensed a strong emotional connection between us and I knew that I was connected to *her* inner emotions.

Within a few minutes her tears subsided, the expression on her face changed and she started to smile, her eyes were still closed at this point and I wondered what she was feeling. I had seen treatments like this before and the outcome was always a revelation, so I would have to wait for her to tell me at the end of the session.

By now she had fallen asleep. It was a shame that I had to disturb her by waking her up from such a peaceful sleep, but as I spoke to her she gently opened her eyes and sat up while I completed my post-treatment notes.

It was now time to get some answers and I was looking forward to asking her how she felt. As she spoke to me her voice was soft and gentle and she chose her words very carefully. She told me that a year earlier, as she went into labour with her first child, the surgeon had opted for a caesarean section. He didn't explain why, but she trusted that there must be a good reason for his decision although she was disappointed. She wanted to be able to watch her child being born and have her husband by her side in the delivery room.

During the procedure, she was experiencing excruciating pain and it was obvious to her that the anaesthesia that was administered was not working. She cried out in pain but no one in the theatre took any notice of her and the only thing that separated her from the surgeons' scalpel was a green sheet that the theatre nurse had put in place. By now, she was terrified and in agony and she couldn't understand why her cries for help were being ignored and giving birth had become her worst nightmare!

Several minutes later, she heard her baby cry and a short time after that her baby daughter was gently placed on her chest. She was a healthy, beautiful baby with a lovely complexion and not a hint of a wrinkle in sight.

At last the surgeon and theatre nurses realized that something was terribly wrong because Jacky began to cry out in pain as the sutures were being put in and Jacky was given more aesthetic. Only then did she feel some relief from the pain. Jackie commented that the delivery of her baby had left a lasting psychological effect on her and she was still having nightmares a year later.

Then she recalled that as soon as I placed my hands on her head at the start of the treatment, she had felt as if I had wrapped her up in a warm blanket. She remembered drifting off into a half-awake, half-asleep kind of consciousness that was very comforting. It was then that the memory of her ordeal came flooding back, only this time her story had a happy ending!

She saw herself lying in the operating theatre, then in an instant, she was standing next to the surgeon on the other side of the sheet watching her baby being delivered and this time she didn't feel any pain at all. When she saw her baby being born, she couldn't hold back the tears of joy and cried at the miracle of it all, then the next thing she remembered was when I placed my hand on her shoulder to wake her up.

Now, she wasn't sure what this all meant because she had just had the same nightmare that she had experienced many times before, but how, and why had her nightmare ended in such a different way? After all, her baby was nearly a year old now so what had brought about the change in her dream, and would this be only a temporary respite from the nightmares that she was having?

This was a lot for her and me to take on board, but I felt sure that Jacky had returned to the dream to be free from the hold that it had on her. Over the next few months when I saw her I always asked her how she was, and she confirmed what I had thought, her repeating nightmare had ended.

CASE STUDY 11: A FLYING FISH IN THE SPA!

'Life force energy' resides in every living thing, including plants, animals and fish!

I arrived for work as usual and was greeted by Jenny, the Spa manager; she was quite upset because her Goldfish had jumped out of its bowl!

We used to have two goldfish in the Spa reception but a few weeks earlier one of them had died. I personally know very little about goldfish but perhaps the surviving fish may have been lonely and had been looking for its companion. Anyway, on this particular morning the fish had jumped out of its bowl and had dropped onto the stone floor. The cleaning lady had witnessed the leap and scooped the fish up as quickly as possible and put it back in the bowl. The problem was that this had happened two hours earlier and since then the fish had lain on its side and was floating on the top of the water.

At this point Jenny asked me if I could give the fish some Reiki and her request was overheard by some of my colleagues who were looking at the Goldfish in the bowl. When they heard Jennies request they all began to smile and I knew what they were thinking. 'How can you give a fish Reiki'? Well, up to this point I had never thought of treating a fish but it was a living creature, with its own life force energy so I thought, why not!

Everyone stood around and watched in anticipation as I placed my hands a few inches away from the sides of the bowl, then a minute or two later something happened. I felt a flood of Reiki energy move into the bowl and I knew that the fish *was* taking Reiki! As we looked on, the fish started to breath normally and after a couple of minutes began to swim in an upright position. Everyone, including me was surprised at what we were seeing and there was such a change in the fish that Jenny dropped a pinch of fish food into the water and it started feeding.

For a week or two after, the fish was perfectly healthy but unfortunately the story has a sad ending because it was found dead on the floor.

CASE STUDY 12: THE BALANCING EFFECTS OF A REIKI TREATMENT

Caroline was suffering from stress, she explained that she had been having I.V.F. - 'In-vitro fertilization' to help her conceive and after 2 failed attempts she felt very stressed about the whole process. She had tried Reiki some years earlier and it had helped with some of her problems then and thought that it might be worth trying again.

She made herself comfortable and I started the treatment. From the outset, she seemed to let go and I had the feeling that she felt very heavy while she was lying there. This might seem like a strange comment to make but sometimes I feel like the person on the couch, when I say 'feel' I mean I have their sensations which can be of a physical, emotional or spiritual nature and this 'lets me know' what my client is feeling.

I began to feel as heavy as a stone, and then my thoughts were somewhere else and I saw a brilliant white light and this meant that Caroline was moving into a heightened state of consciousness and was in a blissful state of relaxation. By the time I reached her feet, which was at the half-way stage she was sound asleep. I gently woke her and asked her to turn over onto her tummy and she quickly fell asleep again and didn't move for the duration of the treatment.

I woke her up at the end to tell her that the treatment was over and she looked very relaxed and peaceful and it was at this point that I asked her how she felt. She said that she had seen lots of images during the treatment but the first one was the best as she had seen a "bright white light." She couldn't tell me at what part of the treatment she had seen it, but she didn't need to, because I had seen it myself, although at this point I didn't tell her what I had seen.

Another thing Caroline mentioned was that after she had seen the 'light', her body had started to 'tingle all over' and she said that it felt like a weak electrical pulse was moving through her body. She commented that it felt "strange but pleasant."

She said that there was something else that was very unusual because she felt like she was being 'pressed down onto the couch.' At one point she wanted to move her arms but felt that she was unable to! Her comments were almost word for word what I had written in my post treatment notes and when I read them to her she was very surprised. At first she thought I had read her mind but I explained that sometimes the energies are so finely tuned between the practitioner and the recipient that the two energies merge to become one.

A month later the Spa was buzzing with people because the Spa director had organized a charity event for 'Breast Cancer awareness week' and the tickets had sold out. The Spa Director had decided to offer 'taster sessions' and my contribution was 'Mini' Reiki treatments lasting fifteen minutes each. The event started at 4pm and by ten past four I had a queue of about twenty people outside my door. I decided to leave the door open as this would give the other guests an opportunity to see what was going on and it would also be interesting for them to see the reactions that others had to the treatment and I could also have 5 guests in my room at the same time which was quite a novelty!

After an hour or so, I saw Caroline who had come for her treatment a month earlier. She was standing in the doorway. I presumed that she was waiting for her turn to have a 'mini' session but as I looked at her, she gave me an amazing smile. She looked much better than when I had seen her a month previously with no signs of the stress that she had, in fact, she looked perfectly brimming with health and it was then that I thought that she might be pregnant, because she looked radiant!

A few minutes past and now she was standing in front of me. She threw her arms around me and told me she was pregnant and we both had tears in our eyes. The other women in the room congratulated us both and it was at this point that I realized that everyone had got the wrong idea; they all thought that I was the father! Then I tried to explain that I was not Caroline's husband and this made everyone even more confused. Caroline interrupted me to put the record straight by explaining about the Reiki treatment that she had received a month earlier and that 'I was only her therapist,' and at that moment everyone fell about laughing.

Caroline told me that when she missed her period, she went to see her Gynaecologist who confirmed that she was pregnant! He said that this should not be possible because he had told her that she would have to wait three months to have another I.V.F treatment because she had such a cocktail of hormones in her system that it would be almost impossible for her to conceive.

When Caroline gave birth to Amy, a healthy baby girl, she and her husband came to my home to show her to me, she was lovely, a beautiful little baby with blond hair and blue eyes. I was so fortunate to have had the opportunity to treat someone in need and I had learnt another valuable lesson from this, Stress prevents us from living a 'normal life.' We should never give up hope, we should try to let go of the negative thoughts that prevent us from living an amazing life, and then just maybe, anything is possible.

CASE STUDY 13: OUR REIKI BABY

Sometimes the things I see are exceptional and it takes a lot of getting used to but I never fail to be in awe at the way Reiki transforms people's lives. Every now and again I get a glimpse of how this Universe of ours works; and this case was another one of those occasions.

A young woman called Mary was waiting to speak to me in the Spa reception. She looked really nervous and when I introduced myself, this didn't help, because she took one look at me and I could see what she was thinking. She looked to be in her mid- twenties and very petite, I on the other hand was built like a Rugby player and I must have looked very intimidating to her. I have to admit that it has been a common misconception with people who meet me for the first time that I am a big, strong man with a bald head and hands the size of dinner plates, "have you got the picture"? Well, I do have all of these physical features but the truth of the matter is that I am 'a gentle giant.'

Mary followed me to my room, sat down and I lowered my voice to a whisper as I asked her to complete a Spa medical questionnaire, and within a minute or two I could feel that she felt more comfortable about having a Reiki treatment with me.

She had not had a Reiki treatment before and didn't even know what the treatment consisted of but it had been recommended to her by one of the other therapists who felt sure that it would help her to relax and ease the stress and tension that she was suffering from.

Due to the volume of treatments that I had done in the past, I had seen some wonderful examples of how a Reiki treatment had helped people who were suffering from stress and I assured her that Reiki could certainly help reduce her stress levels.

I briefly explained the treatment to her and asked her to lie on the Reiki table, with her arms placed by her side. I told her that I was going to play some relaxing music and that she should try not to think about anything and just close her eyes and maybe listen to the music. I was very surprised, because she did just that!

From the outset I knew that something special was going to happen, although I didn't know what it was but I felt a sense of anticipation and a couple of times during the treatment I felt euphoric. I knew from past experience that there was always a reason for what I felt and I was very excited at the prospect of finding out what this was!

I completed my post-treatment notes then asked Mary if she had felt anything from the treatment. Her eyes were opened wide like saucers as she recalled what had happened. She said that she had 'seen a white light' and that it was so bright that she had to keep her eyes tightly closed to prevent it from hurting them and she had the sensation of feeling waves moving over and through her body! She had never experienced anything like this before and she said that it felt so good that she had not wanted the treatment to stop because it had left her feeling totally relaxed, something that she had rarely felt before.

I then tried as best as I could to explain why some people *see* things during their treatments and said that on occasions clients also 'feel things' and this was because they needed to. These feelings and sensations were there to give you exactly what you need - 'Designer medication.'

Mary then asked me a lot of questions about Reiki, she was intrigued and I could tell that she was really taken with her treatment. She wanted to know why I became a Reiki Master and after telling her, I said that I would email her some information about the origins of Reiki etc.

Before she left she told me that they had been trying for a baby for a number of months but had no success and wondered if her treatment might help her to be more relaxed about the whole thing. I said that being stressed about it was definitely not helping and that I felt sure that she would feel much calmer about it.

After she left, a thought crossed my mind. Did I feel euphoric at the beginning of the treatment because my senses knew that she was going to conceive or was there another reason for this feeling?

A few days later her husband George phoned me because Mary had convinced him that they should do the Reiki level 1 course with me, so I offered them a date for the following month.

A couple of weeks passed then George phoned me again only this time he was so excited that I could hardly understand what he was saying. He said that Mary was pregnant and that the doctor had confirmed the date and that their baby was due in early summer and that Mary had conceived on the day of her Reiki treatment, and he wanted to thank me.

I was really pleased for them, and said that he didn't have to thank me because she had let go of her stress and tension during the treatment and maybe that was the reason that she had been unable to conceive before. It was just a case of letting her body relax and balance itself and the treatment had done that for her, not me.

Mary's baby was born in early summer and she was a beautiful little baby girl. She had big brown eyes, lots of hair and was perfect. Mary and George came to visit me a few months later to show me their beautiful daughter and I was delighted to hear them call her their 'Reiki baby,' this is testament to the effects that this wonderful healing energy has on people.

This story is an example of my 'feeling' that 'something special' was about to happen, but not understanding what it was. Fortunately for me, I got to find out, but this has not always been the case because the majority of the clients that I treated in Cyprus were tourists from other countries and I never met them again.

George went on to complete his Reiki level 1 and 2 course and is now well on the way to understanding the joys of being a Reiki practitioner and will be taking his advanced Reiki training and Master-teacher training in 2011.

CASE STUDY 14: A DIFFERENT WAY TO TAKE YOUR REIKI

A treatment comes to mind that was very interesting and it gave me an opportunity to try an alternative method of giving Reiki to someone.

I had just started a Reiki seminar at the Spa where I worked when a Doctor who also worked at the Spa turned up to watch, she was fascinated by what I was doing. I offered to give her a demonstration to enable her to *feel some Reiki,* but she became very nervous and although I felt that she wanted to try it, she declined my offer. A few days later I was running another seminar and the Doctor turned up again only this time she accepted my offer to participate. I explained to the guests that although it appeared that I was here to 'give them some Reiki,' the truth of the matter was that it was impossible for me to impose Reiki on others whether they needed it or not. If they needed some Reiki, they would take it from me.

I asked for a volunteer and the Doctor who I shall call 'Maria' stepped forward and lay down on the table. As I scanned her with my hands, she jolted violently and this made me and the onlookers jump with surprise! I had seen something of a similar nature before but never on someone that I had not even touched. Undeterred, I attempted to place my hands on her head but she jolted again. This was very unusual and it was fascinating to watch but I wanted to find out why this had happened, then a thought crossed my mind. I knew of two other options that I could try to give her a treatment.

The first option was to *send* her some Reiki but I could only do that when I was on my own. The second option was to infuse a bottle of water with Reiki and let her drink the water slowly during the day. The latter option was an excellent way to treat children who were hyperactive; who would not sit still for a treatment and in both instances the patient or client still had the opportunity to refuse permission. This choice of rejecting or accepting the treatment would determine the outcome. Unfortunately the Doctor would not be able to receive her Reiki in the usual way in front of the other guests so later that day I gave her a bottle of Reiki water.

After the seminar, I drew some Reiki symbols over the outside of a bottle of water and then periodically throughout the day placed my hands over the bottle to let Reiki flow into the water. This sounds impossible and I have to say that until I tried some Reiki water myself a few years earlier I didn't really believe that it was possible.

I explained to Maria that she could sip the Reiki water slowly during the day and this would be an excellent way to self-medicate, I also asked her to check the seal on the bottle which she did, to confirm that it was not broken. This was proof that I had not put anything other than Reiki into the water. I said that if the Reiki water didn't have any effect, I could try sending Reiki to her.

A couple of days passed and then Maria came to see me. She looked happy and I guessed that by the look on her face she had not had any adverse reactions to the Reiki water.

She commented that the water had tasted different than normal; she had drunk it slowly during the day as I had suggested and it had made her feel relaxed and calm. She asked me how it was possible to put Reiki into the water without breaking the seal on the bottle so I briefly explained the process to her. She couldn't really grasp the concept but accepted that it had certainly made a difference to how she felt and this had been a pleasant surprise.

At this point I asked her if she would be willing to try some Reiki again in the conventional way and she agreed so I asked her to hold her hands out in front of me. Almost immediately she felt the flow of Reiki in her hands when I placed my hands beneath hers and she could feel tingling sensations in both of them, then the sensations started to move up her arms. I said that the sensations that she was feeling was Reiki moving towards the areas of imbalance and because Reiki was an intelligent energy and knew where her problems were this was completely normal.

Then I moved my hands and placed them close to one of her Chakras, being very careful not to touch it. The Chakra responded by drawing Reiki from my hands and this reassured her that Reiki could do her no harm. At no time during this mini- demonstration did she jolt and I deduce from this that she must have been ultra-sensitive to Reiki on the first occasion and now her body had become de-sensitized or balanced by drinking the water.

This leads me to believe that our sensitivity to Reiki is a reflection of the life or lifestyles that we have, and the ups and downs of our lives affect our psyche. This is mirrored in our energetic body making it ultra-sensitive for some individuals. This sensitivity is not just to Reiki, but to many things such as the food we eat and the environments we live and work in.

CASE STUDY 15: A FAN OF REIKI

I understand how difficult it is for someone to grasp the concept that Reiki, an invisible spiritual energy could be channelled by anyone without any conscious thought or effort. I used to try my hardest to convince everyone that I spoke to about the benefits that they could get from a Reiki treatment or training.

This story is an example of how Reiki can convince someone who has no belief in it what so ever, especially as this person had never even heard of Reiki.

It was a really hot, humid day and my electrician David had just arrived to install a new ceiling fan in my treatment room. As he started to screw the fan to the ceiling he stopped to rub his arm and shoulder and it became obvious that he was experiencing some discomfort, so I asked him what was wrong.

He said that a few weeks earlier he had injured his arm while at work and because he had to work 6 days a week, the injury had not had sufficient time to heal. I asked him if had ever heard of Reiki, he said he had not, so I briefly explained that it was a healing energy that had its origins in Japan and that I was a practitioner. I offered to give him a few minutes of Reiki on his arm and shoulder and he said that he would try anything if it helped with the pain. I asked him if I could draw some Reiki symbols over the painful area. He was a little bemused by this and looked at me as if I was some kind of geek but agreed. I drew the symbols on his arm and shoulder and then placed my hands down then instantly my hands began to tingle and get very hot.

After about 5 or 6 minutes the sensations in my hands subsided so I asked David how his arm felt. At first, he was reluctant to move his arm but slowly and tentatively he flexed the fingers on his right hand and lifted his arm. He then gave me a look of surprise because a few minutes earlier this movement had been excruciatingly painful but now he said there was no pain at all! He couldn't understand this and commented that "Reiki was like magic." "How on earth was this possible" he said? I really didn't have enough time to try and explain how Reiki does this sometimes but said that it's a case of being in the right place at the right time, and he seemed happy with my reply.

I few minutes later, David finished installing the fan and after testing it to make sure it worked thanked me for my help and went on his way, he glanced back at me as he got in his van with a look that I would see on a regular basis from some of my other clients.

CASE STUDY 16: KEEPING PACE

Tom didn't really understand all this 'invisible energy stuff' although he had tried Reiki a few times and it appeared that he got some benefit from his treatments. Petra his wife was a Reiki convert and had booked him a treatment because it would do him good. When she introduced him to me, he informed me that he had been fitted with a heart pacemaker the previous year. I explained to him that Reiki was a form of energy and that this energy might have some impact on his pacemaker! He was very relaxed about the whole thing and said that he had tried 'the occasional' Reiki treatment since having the pacemaker fitted and had not experienced any adverse effects, and was sure he would be ok.

I led him into the treatment room and asked him to complete and sign the medical questionnaire, as this was a declaration of his willingness to have the treatment based on what I had told him. He signed the form, lay on the Reiki table and I asked him to inform me immediately if he began to feel unwell or have any increase in his heartbeat etc. He agreed to do this and I tentatively started the treatment.

This was the first time that I had treated anyone with a heart pacemaker and I must admit to feeling a little nervous, partly because I was a Reiki Master, not a medical professional and due to the nature of his condition, it is always prudent to err on the side of safety when treating someone with a serious heart condition.

I had no need to be concerned because Tom fell asleep after a few minutes and snored loudly every now and again, then as I placed my hands down on his chest, his arms began to lift up off the table and they were still elevated when it was time to move to the next position!

One of the positions in the treatment is done on the palms of the hands; the clients hand is lifted off the table and is then supported by the practitioners so that Reiki may be channelled into the palm chakra. Unfortunately, I couldn't do this hand position with Tom because his hands and arms were now hovering about a foot off the couch, so I just placed my hand beneath his, and carried on with the treatment. By the time I got to his feet, his arms were still in the air and it looked bizarre to say the least to see his arms elevated a foot off the table!

I walked to the head of the table and gently woke Tom from his sleep and asked him to turn over and it was at this point that he saw where his arms were!

He made a comment that it was weird to see his arms up in the air like this and he hadn't a clue why this had happened. I gently motioned his arms back onto the table and asked him to turn over onto his stomach for the second half of the treatment.

The remainder of the treatment was quite uneventful apart from the sound of heavy snoring and at the end of the treatment I woke him to tell him that I had finished.

By now, Tom was calm but confused because he couldn't explain why his arms had risen off the table and said that he had no idea where they were during the treatment. It was at this point that I gave him a glass of water and this gave me time to complete my post treatment notes before I asked him any questions.

With my notes completed, I asked him how he felt. He said that it had been ages since he had slept so well and he didn't want to wake up because he had felt so relaxed and comfortable. He made a comment about his arms being 'Floaty' and said that he had felt them 'doing something' but couldn't stop them lifting off the table! He said that It didn't matter how hard he tried, he couldn't pull them back down again either and It was only when I woke him up and gently motioned them back to the table that they felt *normal* again.

I told him that this sometimes happens, and it was a good indication that he had taken a huge amount of Reiki and it was quite normal. He smiled, and asked me not to tell his wife about what had happened, as he thought she might accuse him of exaggerating. I promised and then we both had a good laugh about it!

I learnt something very important from this treatment because I had read in some Reiki books that it is unwise to treat someone with a heart pacemaker because Reiki may affect the device. I can only speak for myself when I say that on this occasion, the treatment was powerful but extremely gentle and the outcome was that Tom was a very happy client.

Caution should always be exercised when dealing with this kind of device and you should always be informed by the practitioner of any possible risks. Ultimately, if you decide to have a treatment you must sign a declaration to the effect that it is at your own risk and this goes for every client that I treat. Anyone considering having a Reiki treatment should be asked to complete a medical questionnaire by the practitioner before the practitioner agrees to go ahead with the treatment.

A word of caution! If you are not asked to fill in this form it is possible that you are not being treated by a professional Reiki practitioner!

CASE STUDY 17: VOICES FROM THE OTHER SIDE

This next case was bizarre to say the least, but it does show how Reiki can adapt to all kinds of situations.

A guest from the hotel wanted to book a treatment in the Spa but insisted that he needed to speak to me first, so I was called to the reception and introduced to Peter, a middle-aged man. He told me that he had tried Reiki 5 or 6 years ago and that his treatments were very bizarre! He said that during *his* treatments, voices came out of his mouth that were not his own and that they were voices from some of his dead relatives! He went on to describe how he was not in control of what happened during the treatment and said that he wanted to inform me about this strange phenomenon because under these circumstances, I might not want to give him a treatment!

I was intrigued and apprehensive at the same time about what he told me as I had never heard of anyone having a Reiki treatment quite like this before and I was fascinated so I agreed to do the treatment. The truth was that I wanted to find out if the same things would happen during a treatment with me and this would enable me to learn something from the experience.

A few minutes later I started the treatment and almost immediately I felt a strange atmosphere fill the room and I sensed that we were not alone. It felt as if someone or something was watching me, then while my hands were resting on Peter's head, his mouth opened and he started to speak. The voice that came out of his mouth was that of a woman and I listened, spell bound as 'she' spoke!

At this point I wasn't sure if she was speaking to me or to Peter and I was trying to take everything in, just in case I had to repeat what had been said. I was not just a spectator now; I was part of the unfolding mystery and the woman's voice spoke about one of her recently departed relatives who had joined her on 'the other side.' She said that he was OK and that he was with other members of her family and she named some of her family members who had 'passed over' and said that they were very happy to be re-united.

I really couldn't believe how calm I was as I listened to this, I didn't feel nervous or frightened, just excited and the longer the treatment went on, the more bizarre it became!

The voice gave information about someone called David and I gathered that David was not 'dead' because the voice said that David's Passport was due for renewal soon and to tell him to see to it!

Now, this may seem like a very strange way of telling someone that their passport is about to expire but what if this information happened to be true! A little while later another voice started to speak and this time it was that of a middle aged man. He gave some more information which made no sense at all to me, and then the voice changed again to that of an old woman. By the end of the treatment, my head was buzzing, I was trying to remember everything that had been said, and by whom, and by now, I was totally confused. Was I just a bystander, or had I been invited to do the treatment so that I could pass the messages on to Peter? I didn't have to wait long to find out!

I brought Peter a glass of water, completed my notes and then asked him about his treatment but in the back of my mind I was thinking, had he understood and remember the words and sounds that came out of his mouth? When I asked him the question, he said, "I understood everything that was spoken to me." I was so relieved to hear these words that I allowed myself to relax, because during the treatment I had made a conscious effort to keep a mental record of what I had heard! Now Peter could tell *me* what it all meant. What a relief!

I composed myself and waited patiently while he explained who had been 'talking to him'. It was surreal; here I was, listening to someone telling me about how his dead relatives were communicating with him from beyond the grave and some thoughts crossed my mind. Had I really been listening to voices from 'Dead people' or was this just an elaborate hoax for my benefit?

After a while, I made up my mind that this was in fact, 'real' and not a hoax at all, I had been a witness to an amazing treatment, one that I would never forget.

Peter thanked me for my understanding and left the Spa but 5 days later he returned for another session. I was really looking forward to this second treatment and I couldn't help but wonder if it was going to be as remarkable as the first?

I didn't have long to wait to find out and a minute or so into the treatment he started talking again. This time it was with the voice of an old man followed quickly by that of an old lady and I realised that she was talking to me! She called me Philip and spoke to me about things that Peter would have had no knowledge of; some personal things that only my family would have been aware of. This old lady was my grandmother! She had died before I was born and I had no memory of her apart from an old black and white photograph, but what she said to me convinced me that she and he were genuine!

By the time I finished his treatment Peter was sound asleep and I had to wake him up. I asked him to tell me about his treatment and the first thing that surprised him was that this was the first time that he had ever received a message for someone else! He heard everything that had been said but didn't understand who the woman was and it took him completely by surprise when I told him that it was my Grandmother.

Peters' treatment had given *me* an insight into a world that I had not known of before and it was a fascinating experience that I shall remember for a very long time.

CASE STUDY 18: A BIT OF A SCEPTIC

Roxanne was a bit of a sceptic when it came to things like Reiki but decided to try a treatment anyway because she had been to one of my Reiki seminars a few days earlier and had "felt something" unusual. I decided that it would be better for her if I didn't explain what any of the Reiki sensations felt like as this would benefit her more than describing what the common sensations were. I knew that a 'blind treatment' would be the best way to treat her; she agreed and said that it would be interesting to see what she felt.

As I started the treatment, I could feel different sensations in my hands; sometimes they would "tingle," and then they would get very hot or even cold. When I got to her hands, I lifted one of them off the table and placed my hand beneath it so that her hand was now resting on my palm. Within a second or two her hand started to lift up from mine and it stopped a foot or so up in the air and just "hovered." I left my hand resting on the couch for a few minutes because I could feel her hand drawing Reiki from mine.

I walked around to the other side of the table, lifted her other hand and placed my hand beneath this one and the same thing happened. When the sensations in my hands subsided I moved on to her knees and only then did her hands move slowly back down onto the table.

After I had finished the treatment I asked her what she had felt. She said that she was very surprised to feel the sensations that had moved through her body and she couldn't wait to tell me! She said that when I first placed my hands on her head, she felt something like an electric current flow through her head and travel all the way down to her feet. It was a very pleasant sensation that had the effect of relaxing the whole of her body, including her mind and she said that from that moment on, her thoughts had just 'disappeared.' It felt very liberating.

She also told me that she could feel my hands on her clothes from time to time but sometimes it felt like more than one pair of hands! I pointed out that this is a common occurrence for some clients, as was the lifting of the hands from the table, although she had not done it intentionally. "Why", she said, "did my hands and arms seem to have a will of their own? I have to admit it felt wonderful, like a kind of floating sensation in my hands and all over my body."

She was so overwhelmed by how light she felt during the treatment because there was a time when she couldn't even feel herself touching the table, and said that she was not asleep and had definitely not dreamt it.

Roxanne had experienced some wonderful sensations from her treatment and I should think that having a Reiki treatment would be a regular occurrence for her in the future.

CASE STUDY 19: JOHNS' WEIRD TREATMENT

I have been very fortunate to do several thousand treatments over the years and some of these were very 'unusual' to say the least, here is one that I hope you will find interesting.

John had not experienced a treatment before so I asked him to complete a medical questionnaire before starting the treatment. I explained that I would start the first hand placements on his head and would move slowly down his body until I reached his feet and this would take approximately thirty minutes. I would then ask him to turn over and continue with the second half of the treatment, finishing at his feet for the second time. If he fell asleep I would gently wake him and he could then make himself comfortable while I completed my post-treatment notes and once I had completed these he might want to give me some feedback or ask some questions.

As soon as I started the treatment I felt some sensations in my hands; it was like a kind of mild electric current, similar to static electricity. Then I noticed that John's arms began to lift off the table and were raised a few inches! It appeared to me that his arms were as light as a feather because there was no sign of tension in them but it looked very strange with his arms floating in mid-air! His arms remained elevated and when I reached his feet I asked him to turn over so that I could start the second half of his treatment. John then opened his eyes and he looked very surprised to see his hands up in the air! He commented that he knew his hands had 'floated away' but as hard as he had tried, he couldn't pull them back down onto the table!

It was now time for him to turn over onto his front so that I could I start the second half of the treatment and again the same thing happened. Within a minute or so, his hands lifted up off the table but this time they moved sideways and his arms were now a long way up in the air. He lay motionless, showing no signs of tension in his body and he remained this way while I completed the treatment.

Now I had to move his out-stretched arms back to the sides of his body before I could walk past them and I couldn't help noticing how light they felt.

I poured John a cool glass of water and asked him to lie there for a few minutes until I had completed my notes. When I asked him for his comments the first thing that he said was that the treatment seemed to be over in no time at all and another weird thing was that it felt like I was moving around the table very fast; almost as if time had been 'speeded up.' He said that something else had happened as I placed my hands over his eyes. He tried to explain his experience by saying that although his eyes were closed, he had seen an intense bright light that had almost blinded him. The light was brighter than anything he had ever seen before and... it was purple!

I knew that John had 'seen something' because I had felt his eyelashes flicker beneath my fingers, something that had happened on many occasions before with other clients. It meant that Reiki had expanded his consciousness.

John then brought up the question of his arms and hands. "They seemed to have a will of their own!" he said. "It was as if my arms were as light as a feather and I had no control of what they were doing." He also asked me if I had seen this happen before and I said that I had, on a few occasions.

The result of this treatment was that John was now feeling totally relaxed and he said that he felt an inner calmness that he had not felt for a long time. He described it as a kind of 'inner peace'. He asked me how long this feeling would last. I told him that sometimes the benefits of a treatment may last a few days, weeks or even months and I recommended that he should keep a journal for the next few days to remind him of the benefits that he had noticed.

CASE STUDY 20: A NEW GIFT FROM REIKI

I had been a practicing full-time Reiki Master-Teacher for a few years when I had a remarkable experience that changed my perception of 'energy.' I was doing lots of treatments at the time and this day had started just like any other, or so I thought!

I worked in a Spa that had a relaxation area where clients wait for their therapists to collect them. On this particular day I noticed a group of 4 or 5 women chatting to each other when one woman caught my eye. Although she was talking to another woman and smiling, I sensed a feeling of great sadness emanating from her. This was a an unusual feeling for me because I always feel positive and I needed to know if what I sensed about her was real or just my imagination.

My hands were starting to get very hot and 'tingle' just like the sensations that I get when I do my treatments. I had also felt these sensations many times before when I demonstrated Reiki during some of my seminars. During these seminars I didn't touch the participants because I wanted the clients to 'feel' or 'sense' the energy that was flowing from me. This gave me an opportunity to judge for myself what was happening. The unusual thing now was that I was not even thinking about Reiki but my inner emotions were letting me know that this woman was feeling sad.

I offered to top up the ladies' water glasses and when I came to the 'sad woman' she briefly looked up at me, and then in an instant she burst into tears!

I could see that she felt embarrassed, so I took her to my treatment room. Once inside she asked me, "Why when I looked at you did I have an overwhelming urge to cry"? I knew the answer! I told her that sometimes just being in the same room as a Reiki practitioner is enough to release the emotional tension from someone and it was at this point that I told her that I had felt her emotional state, although I was not 100% sure of my feelings.

She proceeded to tell me that the previous 6 months of her life had been awful, the worst time of her life and she said that "anything that could have gone wrong did," This had left her feeling totally drained.

Within a few minutes she had composed herself and I recommended that if she had time, she should have a Reiki treatment because she really needed to release the emotional tension that had built up inside her.

This was the first time that my senses had been so acute and I wondered if this was a one-off, but during the day, I did 3 treatments and in every instance I knew what my client's emotional state was, it was as if I had some kind of invisible link or connection to each of them and now I knew that my feelings *were* correct!

I use the word 'feelings' loosely here because at no time was I focusing or thinking about my clients' emotional state, it had just happened. Overnight I had developed an acute sense of awareness that enabled me to feel what my clients were feeling, I could not however read their minds and I was relieved about that because this would have been an intrusion of their privacy.

Over the next few weeks, I learnt how to deal with problems that were not visible by sight, but I knew they were there because I could feel them. They were tangible and I used Reiki symbols to treat them. Sometimes I would feel the emotional pain from a client and would do an 'emotional healing' on them. Each time I chose to use the symbols for this purpose I saw a dramatic change in my clients' condition and it was always a positive improvement.

Reiki had 'upgraded' me and this enabled me to treat many more people in a way that was less intrusive because I didn't have to ask any of them what they were feeling, I could feel for myself.

CASE STUDY 21: LOVE FROM AN UNBORN CHILD

It has been my good fortune to experience many remarkable treatments and this next treatment was one of them.

Clare was 6 months pregnant and apart from a little backache was in perfect health.

After perusing the Spa menu, she was advised to have either a pre-natal treatment which was gentle and very relaxing, or a Reiki treatment because both had no contra-indications and were suitable for a mum to be.

The last time she had tried a Reiki treatment was 2 years earlier and she had really enjoyed it. She asked if there was any possibility that Reiki may harm her baby and I reiterated what the receptionist had told her earlier that Reiki is "taken" by her and could not possibly harm her or her baby. She was pleased to hear this and after completing the medical questionnaire settled down on the Reiki table.

From the outset, a 'feeling' of calmness filled the room and I knew that this was from the effect of the energy that was flowing and within a few minutes Clare was fast asleep. I had felt this calmness on many occasions when treating pregnant women and I came to the conclusion that the energy was being regulated by the unborn child because, it too, was taking Reiki during the treatment.

To understand this, imagine the feeling you get when you walk into a maternity ward in a hospital. As you enter the room where the babies are sleeping, there is a feeling of calmness and gentleness. These feelings are the same ones that I get when I treat someone who is pregnant; it is tangible and definitely real.

By now the first half of the treatment was over so I asked Clare to sit on the end of the table for the second half so that I could 'sandwich' her between my hands. This is a way of treating someone who cannot lie on their stomach or is in the mid-to late stages of pregnancy.

I now placed one hand on her brow and the other one on the corresponding point at the back of her head and instantly I felt the weight of her body relax as she leant against me. She started to smile at this point and her breathing deepened as she became increasingly more relaxed. I knew that she was feeling the flow of Reiki that was being drawn into her body.

The first half of the treatment had felt wonderful for her and as I slowly and methodically moved my hands from one position to another in the second half Clare began to smile again. I didn't speak to her though because it was obvious that she was really enjoying the treatment and by the time I had finished she was nearly asleep again but sitting up!

I sat her down on a chair, gave her a glass of water, completed my notes and then asked her how she felt. Her eyes began to fill with tears as she described what had happened. She said that she felt she was being surrounded by a warm loving energy that seemed to move over her body like a gentle wave.

As the treatment progressed all she could think of was her baby. She said that it was strange, but wonderfully comforting at the same time and she commented that as my hands moved from one position to another, she had seen lovely pastel colours, although her eyes were closed at the time.

This treatment was by no means unusual as I have seen this phenomenon before but the gentle feelings that permeate the room are a remarkable experience, and I would always recommend a Reiki treatment during pregnancy for this reason alone.

CASE STUDY 22: DOES SCIENCE HAVE AN ANSWER?

Sometimes I meet people whose lives are perceived through scientific eyes and James was one of these, I had treated his wife Penny on a couple of occasions and had met him once or twice when he came to collect her at the end of her treatment.

A few weeks past then out of the blue, Penny asked me if I would teach her Reiki. She was fascinated by the experiences that she had had from her treatments. James on the other hand had never tried Reiki before but because of what his wife had told him, he was intrigued and wanted to "work out" what Reiki was for himself.

So, it was decided, they would both do the course but attend on separate days, this was because Penny didn't want James to try to influence what she was feeling, sensing or thinking about Reiki. I was happy to do this and suggested that if she attended the course first, she should keep a record of her experiences and not tell James anything until he had done his the following week. They both thought that this was a good idea and a couple of weeks later Penny did her course.

A week later, James arrived for *his* course. None of the students had tried a Reiki treatment and I felt that this would be an ideal opportunity to see how they reacted to the attunement process. I wanted this course to be informative, but I also decided that I would not discuss what Reiki was or what might be felt from the attunement process. On this occasion I would just 'do it' and let the students make up their own minds.

I started by giving a brief history of Mikao Usui and the story of how Reiki was discovered in Japan and I then went straight to the first part of the attunement. I was very careful not to mention any of the things that are sometimes felt from the process. Generally, I go into more detail before starting the attunements, but this time I wanted James to be unaware because only then would he truly 'discover' Reiki for himself.

I completed the first part of their attunement without speaking, and then offered everyone a glass of water. I asked them one at a time if they had any experiences to share with the group and I started by asking James if he had felt anything from the attunement process. I said that if he had felt nothing, it was ok to say so because it was good to hear everyone's comments and points of view.

James was surprised because he had seen something when I drew the Reiki symbols over his energy centres.

At the start of the attunement, I had drawn and blown some symbols into his head and as I blew the symbols in, he saw something, although his eyes were closed at the time and this he said had surprised him. He had also *felt* something moving into his body he said when I did a technique called 'The Violet Breath technique' on him. I had not explained this process to him and when I drew another symbol over his 'third eye,' he actually saw an eye! He said that it was as if the eye was looking directly at him and he could clearly *see it!*

He couldn't explain what he had just experienced in scientific terms but he was sure that it had happened. By late morning, I had done the second part of the attunement and all of the students had experienced some sensations or reactions.

After lunch I showed them all a technique called 'Byosen Reikan Ho,' also known as 'body scanning.'

After everyone had tried this, I asked for a volunteer to lie on the couch and James stepped forward. I proceeded to scan his body to 'feel or sense' any imbalances that he might have. I found two areas that took a lot of Reiki and kept a mental record of where they were, then asked each student in turn to scan him and write down on a piece of paper any areas of his body that they felt were imbalanced. I also asked them not to show each other their findings, as we would be putting their findings to the test later.

With our 4 scans completed I told everyone where I had felt the areas of imbalance and then asked them to reveal what they had written in their notes. The other students had 'felt something' in the same places as I did and their notes confirmed this. They were all very surprised and I guess a little relieved at this, but the best was yet to come.

At this point, I explained to James that I may be able to help with these imbalances by drawing some Reiki symbols over these areas; I would then place my hands on them to see what happened.

He was surprised that everyone had located where his problems were and agreed to let me draw the symbols on these areas. He said that he preferred not to see me drawing the symbols; this was because he wanted to see if he would feel anything from the process. So, before I started to draw the symbols on him, I asked him to close his eyes.

I drew the first symbols over his sacral chakra or tanden; this is an area approximately 3 inches below the navel. Just as I finished drawing them James shuddered. Everyone saw that it was precisely as I finished drawing the symbol and they were really surprised. James made a comment that up to this point he had felt something building up inside him and that *something* had moved down his body, but he couldn't explain what that something was.

It was now time to place my hands down where I had drawn the symbols and there was an instant channelling of Reiki energy into the area. I felt a tremendous rush of heat in my hands at this point and I thought that it might be interesting to let one of the other students put his hands there for a minute or two to see what he could feel. I asked Tom, one of the other students if he would like to feel what was happening, he placed his hands down and straight away he felt a huge rush of something in his hands. That 'something' was Reiki being channelled and after 4 or 5 minutes his sensations subsided. For the second time, James had the sensation of something building up inside his body and then being released down his legs.

I knew that this meant that the imbalance was 'fixed' or at the very least would be much better. I now turned my attention to his knees, the other area of imbalance that I had sensed, and drew some more symbols over them too. The same thing happened again and James shuddered once more. Again, I asked Tom to place his hands palms down onto the knees to let Reiki flow into them. He was really surprised because he could feel the flow of energy in his hands and it felt unusual; because he didn't really expect to be able to feel anything from *his* hands.

By now, Tom was feeling a build-up of energy in his hands which came to a peak and then subsided. When he told me this I explained that this was the sensations of 'a Reiki cycle,' and being able to feel this from his hands was an indication that he was sensitive to Reiki and a good channel for the energy.

As the flow of Reiki peaked, James had felt it surge as it travelled down his legs and out through his feet once more and this was what caused him to shudder. After 4 or 5 minutes Tom said that his hands now felt different, more 'normal' so I asked James to sit up so that he could tell us what he had felt. As he sat up he gave me 'that look,' the one that I see from time to time that says, "I don't understand how this can be but I have no signs of the problem."

I asked James to get off the treatment table and he stood up and told us that years ago when he was a young man he had injured his lower back in an accident. He said that he had been in pain ever since but now, unbelievably; he had no signs of the pain at all and was astonished by what had just happened!

After all, he hadn't told us where his problems were, but we had all been able to find where they were located and that had really impressed him.

He said that his knees felt much better and again, he hadn't told us about those either, so although he couldn't work out how Reiki had done it, he knew that Reiki had, and there was a difference in his physical condition to prove it!

I felt that now was a good time to ask the other students' if they had experienced or felt anything from their hands when they had 'scanned' James and it became obvious that everyone had felt something. For the most part, no one could easily describe the sensations that were coming from their hands during the scan but this was quite normal, although this is of little use when you are trying to describe how Reiki works to others.

It is extremely difficult to describe an attunement, I know because I have trained many students and when I ask them to interpret what had just taken place they struggle to find the words to describe their feelings and sensations, this is because every attunement and student is different.

It has been a few years since James had his attunement and he still has no problems in his lower back, but his knees still give him pain from time to time.

Recently, I ran a Reiki 1 class and two of the students that attended had almost identical visual experiences from their attunements. This phenomenon had never happened before, maybe this was because the students were 'in tune' with each other energetically? Anyway, this is their account of what happened.

I had just completed the first part of the attunement and asked the students if they had felt or experienced anything. Robert the first student said that he had *seen* a Pyramid and that I was standing next to it. When I asked his partner Monika she said that she had seen the same thing! This was very unusual, so I asked them both in turn to describe in more detail the images that they had seen and this time there were some slight differences.

Firstly, Robert said that the Pyramid that he had seen was in the distance, and I was standing in the foreground with the Pyramid a long way behind me, Monika on the other hand said that I was dwarfed by the size of the Pyramid that I was standing next too, so although they had both seen me in their images, what they were describing was indeed their own image and interpretation of that image. The strange thing here was that they both saw a Pyramid and they both saw me in their images! Now, if I asked a statistician what the odds would be of 2 people having this kind of recollection, I am sure it would be highly unlikely.

I know that there is always an element of trust involved when you ask people questions, because you may not always get a truthful answer, but experience told me that these students were both telling the truth.

Robert went on to complete his Master/Teacher training with me before I left Cyprus in 2010 and Monika has now done her second course.

CASE STUDY 23: SCIENCE HAS ONLY SOME OF THE ANSWERS FOR NOW!

This case is about a scientist who works with, and measures energy.

Gale had been a scientist all her life and I first met her in the spring of 2009 when she booked a couple of Reiki treatment at the Spa where I worked.

Both of Gales' treatments had given her something to think about because she had felt *something* other than the warmth of my hands on her clothes and this intrigued her.

Her holiday came to an end and she returned home, but a couple of weeks later she emailed me to ask if I could recommend anyone who could give her a treatment or teach her Reiki in the area where she lived.

I said that unfortunately I didn't know of anyone personally, but she should try the internet as a first port of call or her local press. A couple of weeks went by and she sent me another email and this time she said that she was interested in learning Reiki and would be willing to return to Cyprus for the training if I would teach her. I sent her some pre-course information and a short time later she returned to do the Reiki level 1 course with me.

On the day of the course I had to recruit the help of Sandra, one of my students to help with the practical sessions, because the other student who had booked to do the course had been told that she had to work at the last minute.

The morning was taken up with the first and second parts of the attunement and Gale experienced quite a few sensations from these. Now it was time for the practical sessions so I demonstrated how to give a Reiki treatment to herself, a short treatment on someone else and finally the hand positions for a full body treatment.

I showed Gale how and where she should place her hands to give a full body hands-on treatment on Sandra and then it was Gales' turn to give Sandra a treatment.

From the start, Gale could feel the flow of energy in her hands but she also felt something else and commented that her hands felt like she was *giving* and *receiving* Reiki at the same time. It was at this point that Sandra said that as soon as Gale had placed her hands on her, *she* had felt *her* hands heat up and was channelling Reiki into Gale.

What was happening was that Gale the level 1 student was channelling Reiki into Sandra the Reiki 2 student and Sandra was unintentionally channelling Reiki back into Gale, although the treatment was being performed by Gale. This dual flow of Reiki from one person to another was created by Gale's need and this was an excellent example of how Reiki has its own intelligence because it will always flow to where it is needed.

CASE STUDY 24: ARTHRITIC KNEES

Cathy had recently undergone surgery on both of her knees. There had been signs of wear and tear for a number of years and to complicate matters she also had painful Arthritis.

I knew from previous experience that when treating anyone with a painful condition there can sometimes be an increase in pain during the treatment. I started by placing my hands on her head and she commented that her knees were "getting hot" and I knew that Reiki had travelled straight to where the problem was and this excited me because this was an indication that the painful condition that she was suffering from was being rapidly healed.

A treatment like this one has huge benefits for the patient, and the practitioner may be able to see the results before the patient has even got off the table! As soon as I had finished the treatment, Cathy who was feeling very calm now commented that she couldn't feel any pain in her knees and she was very relieved. Now I know that this sounds too good to be true but some of the results that Reiki gives are nothing short of a "Miracle," and on other occasions they can be mediocre. Unfortunately, this has very little to do with the practitioner; and more to do with the clients' needs and wishes.

I have experienced many remarkable healings but if you were to ask me to give you a treatment like the one I gave your friend it would not be possible. This is because *you* take what *you* need, not what the practitioner decides to give you. The practitioner is just a channel for the energy and has very little choice about the outcome of the treatment. Personally, I feel that it is a good idea to have some expectations of what benefits you would like to get from your treatment before you have it, but you should be realistic, if the outcome of your treatment was up to the practitioner, then everyone would be healed but unfortunately, not everyone wants to be healed although they may say they do.

CASE STUDY 25: RAPID HEALING

Pauline had been having gynaecological problems for a while and her consultant decided that it would be in her best interests to have a hysterectomy. I had only met her on a couple of occasions before and because she was living in England I offered to send her some distant healing, before, and after the surgery. Her husband said that he would let me know how she was doing and would inform me if she felt anything from the distant healing.

The day after her surgery I sent her a thirty minute treatment and later that day I received an email to say that she was recovering well after the surgery. The following day a second email arrived to say that the surgeon was surprised at how quickly she was recovering and that she would probably be able to leave the hospital 5 days later, but on the third day, I received another email to say that she had been allowed home. The surgeon and her husband were both amazed at the rapid healing that had taken place in such a short period of time because it had only been three days since her surgery. I have found from my experiences that it is not uncommon to have a rapid healing after having a Reiki treatment, and the incidence of post-treatment infection is reduced because there is no need to touch your patient when administering the treatment.

CASE STUDY 26: A NATURAL BALANCE

Ann was a therapist who came to speak to me about a personal problem. She had been suffering from acne for a while and her doctor had recommended that she take the contraceptive pill to balance her hormones and she was assured that this would clear the acne.

The medication had been very effective but unfortunately, it left her with another problem! She had stopped taking the pill 6 months ago and had not had a period since and she wondered if Reiki might be able to reinstate her periods, she said that not having them made her feel less than a woman. I suggested that she try one treatment initially to see what effect it had but felt sure that this might be a natural way to balance her monthly cycles. I explained that Reiki does have a very balancing effect on the body, including the endocrine- (hormone) system and although there might be more than one cause for her lack of periods, it was certainly worth trying a session. She agreed and the following day she came to me for her treatment. I started the session by scanning her with my hands and as I reached her sacral chakra- an area approximately 3 inches below the navel; I felt a huge amount of energy flowing from my hands.

This area is where the Ovaries are located and this confirmed to me that there was some imbalance there.

I must add at this juncture that even if there is an indication of an imbalance, it would not be wise or correct of me to make a diagnosis, only a physician or a medically trained professional should do this.

A couple of weeks later Pauline informed me that she had started her period and said that she felt relieved and surprised at how quickly the treatment had worked, given the fact that there were no drugs involved.

This was the first time that I had treated anyone with this type of hormone imbalance and it had shown me that a Reiki treatment can work to balance the body in ways that are not fully understood by medical science.

Reiki is a developing therapy and even as we speak, new information and techniques are being found; and some of this information is coming from Reiki practitioners. The sharing of this information is vital to the development of Reiki in the future especially for those Reiki professionals who work full-time and this is another reason that I decided to write this book.

In January 2009 I went to Florida for a holiday and what I found there surprised me.

I bought a health and wellbeing magazine in a local store and as I flicked through the pages I was astonished to see how many hospitals, clinics and doctors' surgeries were offering Reiki to their patients. I hadn't realized how huge Reiki was in Florida!

I decided to go on-line to see if this was the same in the other states and I found that a number of hospitals were also using Reiki therapists and they were treating everything from Migraine headaches to terminal Cancer and I found this extremely encouraging. Unfortunately this does not seem to be the case in other countries as the rest of the world is lagging behind.

I feel that we should treat our illnesses and diseases in the most gentle and cost effective way, this could be with a combination of conventional medicine, complementary medicine and anything else that is effective. Patients are dying every day because of money, or the lack of it and it cannot be right that only those who are able to pay for their medication receive care. Excellent healthcare should be available to those in need irrespective of whether they can afford to pay for it or not and the spiralling costs of drugs, healthcare and private medical insurance around the world makes Reiki a viable option. It is my belief that by using Reiki therapy, our lives will be enriched in so many ways and the use of drugless medicine appears to be on the increase. One reason for this is that there are no side effects from a Reiki treatment, only after- affects and these are generally of a positive nature and do not affect the health of the patient.

Case study 27: The Reiki / Yoga connection

Amy was a woman in her prime; she practiced Yoga and Meditation and enjoyed every minute of her life. She had only tried Reiki once before and was fascinated by what I had told her so she booked a treatment with me. She checked in at the reception desk and I led her to my room and after asking her some relevant questions she made herself comfortable on the table.

Everyone would want a life like Amy's because she had no signs of stress or tension in her body and she was vibrant and full of life and I could sense her life force energy. This was a clear indication of a very happy soul. As I placed my hands on her shoulders to make a connection with her energy, her legs and feet started to rise off the table and when I placed my hands over her Third eye, her head began to push my hands upwards, and a minute later her body was bent upwards in a 'V' shape, with only her bottom touching the table. I was astounded by what I was seeing and noticed that at no time during the treatment did she show any signs of tension in her abdomen, or anywhere else in her body! This was weird, after all, I was looking at a woman whose body was bent almost double and she was totally relaxed, in fact she was so relaxed that she twitched every now and again and I swear that she was falling asleep!

I carried on with the treatment and periodically Amy's body would move into another strange position, then a thought crossed my mind. Was it possible that she was practicing Yoga while she was asleep and if so, why would she do this?

By the time I finished the treatment there were lots of questions going through my mind and now, hopefully, I would find some answers! I asked Amy what sensations she had felt during the treatment and her reply took me by surprise. She commented that she had never experienced anything like this before, and it felt like the treatment had given her a workout. The Reiki treatment had manipulated her body into the Yoga positions, but the sensations that she felt were completely different than when she had practiced Yoga in a class. During this treatment her body had moved effortlessly. She said that there was a time when she became aware that her body was moving but hadn't realized just how much. I had watched in amazement and presumed that she was doing this herself but I had got it totally wrong. Was she awake or asleep during the treatment? I had to know, so I asked her and she said that she was not awake or asleep but was somewhere in between. She could hear the music in the room but was not in control of the movements of her body and was very surprised that the treatment had turned out like this, and said that it felt wonderful.

I had never seen a Reiki treatment quite like this one before but within a couple of months, I encountered another one that was almost identical.

CASE STUDY 28: A TRULY AMAZING EXPERIENCE!

Once in a while, I get to see something very special; and this treatment was exceptional!

Jenny had attended one of my Reiki seminars and a few days later she decided to book a treatment. Her appointment was scheduled for 4.30 pm and at 4.50 pm she came rushing in looking very hot and flustered. She kept apologizing for being late and I told her not to worry because her treatment was the last one of the day and I could take as much time as I wanted without fear of keeping anyone else waiting. I gave her a cool glass of water until she had calmed down and then I started her treatment.

As soon as I placed my hands down on her shoulders she began to laugh and it was then that I noticed her arms and legs were not touching the table and neither was her head! I placed my hands on her head now with my fingers resting on her cheeks and her head began to push my hands up in the air! I thought how strange this was, then Jenny spoke to me, she said, "Can I ask you a strange question"? I said yes and she asked me if her body was touching the table as she couldn't feel the table beneath her! At the time, I thought thank god that she asked the question because now I could explain what was happening to her. I told her that there was a space between her body and the table and she was "hovering in the air." I then asked her if she would like to open her eyes and take a look! I lifted my hands gently away from her head and she slowly lifted her head to take a look for herself, "Oh my God" she said, as she looked down the length of her body towards her feet! The sight of seeing her body floating in mid-air was too much for her to take in and she started to laugh uncontrollably and almost fell off the table! I had seen something similar a few times before but this was usually a few minutes into the treatment, but on this occasion Jenny was wide awake and I had only just started the treatment.

At this point I wondered what would happen if I moved my hands completely away from her body, there was only one way to find out so I asked her if I could take my hands away to see what would happen and she agreed. I thought that as soon as I moved my hands away she might just drop back down on to the table so very slowly I took my hands away and her body slowly and gently settled back down onto the table. Wow, how amazing was that! By now there were lots of thoughts going through my mind and I wondered why this treatment was so unusual, was it something that I had done differently that made this happen or was there another explanation?

Jenny was very surprised to say the least at what was happening and asked me if this was *normal*, I told her that I had experienced a few treatments that were similar and that she could relax and just allow her body to do whatever it wanted and I explained that Reiki has its own intelligence and it knew what kind of treatment she needed to have. She seemed happy with my answer, although she didn't know what to expect next but that made it even more exciting. I continued with the treatment and put my hands back on her head and straight away she lifted off the couch once more and this time her arms and legs were 6 inches in the air! Then her arms began to move sideways, then backwards towards the top of her head!

She then put the palms of her hands together behind her head and placed the pads of her thumbs onto her 'Third eye.' What happened next took her completely by surprise and she said "Wow"! I could tell from the tone of her voice that something had startled her and I said that she could tell me what had happened at the end of the treatment.

As I moved my hands from one position to another the treatment became more and more bizarre because Jenny's arms were constantly 'on the move.' Some of the movements were being repeated over and over again and periodically she spoke to me and said "My hands and arms seem to have a will of their own." And I thought how strange this looked at the time, then her feet and legs lifted up and her legs parted, then the soles of her feet came together and were drawn up towards her groin and they moved downwards again until she almost did the 'Splits' with her legs!

I have to say at this point that Jenny was a little over weight and I thought how supple she was to be able to move her limbs in such a way, she made it look effortless.

By now, neither of us could contain ourselves any longer and we both burst out laughing, the atmosphere in the room was electric and it felt like we were in another dimension, like 'Alice in Wonderland,' only this was for real!

I completed the first half of the treatment and it was time for Jenny to turn over onto her tummy and as soon as I placed my hands on her shoulders again, her arms began to lift off the table once more. Then they moved sideways and she placed her hands on the back of her neck and started to massage it! *My* hands were now 'in the way,' so I moved them and a minute or two later, her hands moved once more and came to rest on the sides of her temples where she started to 'massage' them. She was now 'giving herself a massage.' Now some thoughts crossed my mind, "Who was doing this treatment,"? was it Jenny, Reiki, or me? As I watched in awe as the treatment unfolded I didn't have long to wait before I got some answers.

Jenny's eyes were closed and I knew that she couldn't see where *my* hands were but not once did her hands bump into mine and this led me to believe that either her hands could sense where mine were, or her Third eye was directing the movements of her arms.

Very slowly Jenny's arms moved back by her sides and then her head and legs lifted off the table once more until her body was now in a 'V' shape, I recognized this position from a treatment with someone else and there were other similarities too. On both occasions neither of the clients had shown any tension as their bodies moved into some extremely awkward positions. I remembered at this point that my other client had practiced Yoga and meditation for a number of years and I wondered if Jenny had learnt Yoga and was having some kind of 'guided treatment.' Both women had responded in a similar fashion to the Reiki energy and the movements they did were almost identical and I thought that this might be a common denominator. And, hopefully I would be able to ask a few relevant questions at the end of the treatment to find out.

With the treatment over, I asked Jenny to make herself comfortable while I completed her post-treatment notes and it was then that she looked at me in total disbelief! She had a huge smile on her face and burst out laughing again and I followed suit!

I was sure that everyone had heard us laughing and I wondered what they must be thinking because this was a Spa, a place of quiet relaxation and tranquillity and here we were, laughing uncontrollably.

Words are not enough to explain what had just happened and now it was time for Jenny to tell me about her treatment! "Where do I start" she said, "Let's start at the beginning" I replied.

"The first hand placement was on your brow chakra" I said, "what did you feel when I placed my hands there"? "It felt amazing" she said, "my body instantly felt weightless, as though I was floating on a cloud." She said that it was at this point that I asked you if I was still 'on the table' and I remembered everything that happened although I'm not sure why these things happened. She continued by saying that when she had looked at herself floating in mid-air she couldn't believe her eyes because she was wide awake and definitely not dreaming it, but was this really possible?

I told her that there can be many things in our lives that appear to be 'not possible' but the truth is that they *are* possible, and this was one of them.

Jenny then went on to describe what she had 'seen.' She said that when her hands reached up to her brow, she had not been in control of them at all. It felt like they had a will of their own and when her thumbs touched her Third eye she *saw* a 'bright light' that exploded into hundreds of tiny pieces like an amazing firework display. Her eyes were closed at the time so how could she see?

I now understood what her hands had done. They had opened her third eye and this had expanded her consciousness and had given her a new sensory awareness.

I explained to Jenny that *her* Reiki treatment had also given her a physical workout! She said that she could hardly believe how her body had stretched and been so supple and said that she had not done any of the movements with her body voluntarily; her body had done it of its own volition. It had felt weird and wonderful and while this was happening, she had felt no pain or discomfort and had not even got out of breath!

It was at this point that I decided to ask her how long she had been practicing Yoga because I had seen people practicing yoga in various Spas and had recognized some of the movements that she had been doing. After listening to my comments, she started to laugh again and said "do I really look as if I practice Yoga"?

"I have never been to any kind of fitness class in my life before, let alone Yoga." This really surprised me and then I realized that there must be a link between Yoga and Reiki as I had seen 2 other treatments where the clients had done identical Yoga body movements. These individuals had not met each other but for some reason, both of them had been 'given' a Reiki treatment that included a Yoga workout and this fascinated me!

CASE STUDY 29: 'FIXING' A PERSONAL TRAINER

My next client was a personal trainer who had recently undergone keyhole surgery for a cartilage problem on his knee. Two weeks had passed since the operation and he was still experiencing some pain so I asked him if he would like to try some Reiki on it as it might help with the pain. Bob had not tried Reiki before although he knew a little about it because he worked in the gym that was in the Spa where I worked and had seen me doing Reiki seminars from time to time.

I briefly explained that I was going to draw some Reiki symbols over the front and the back of his knee if that was OK. He agreed, and after I had finished drawing the symbols I placed one hand on the front of his knee and the other on the back of his knee to see what happened. Immediately, I felt a rush of energy into the palms of my hands and this was a sure sign that whatever was causing the pain in his knee was being 'fixed.' I had experienced this energy 'rush' in my hands many times before and the outcome of the treatment was always the same. Whatever the problem was, it would be 'fixed.' I left my hands in place until the sensations subsided and then took them away. From start to finish this had taken just seven minutes.

I asked Bob how his knee felt now and he replied that "it felt Strange." He said that since the surgery he had been in pain but that it now felt 'normal.' He was sitting on my Reiki table so I suggested that he stand up and put some weight on his leg to see how that felt. He stood up and commented that he still couldn't feel any pain. Then he stooped down and flexed his knee, and he still couldn't feel any pain!

Bob was a highly qualified personal trainer and teacher; his business consisted of teaching and training other students to become personal trainers. His knowledge of human anatomy was excellent, and he knew that it was necessary to have the surgery on his knee. One thing that he couldn't understand however was that his knee was now pain free and I had only put my hands on it for a few minutes.

The following morning I asked him how his knee was, he said that his knee was fine and he was really surprised by the outcome of the treatment.

CASE STUDY 30: THE GIFT OF LIFE

Susan came to me because she was suffering from depression and was desperate to try anything that might help. I handed her a medical questionnaire to fill in, she paused for a moment to read it and asked why I needed to know if she had undergone any surgery in the last three years. I said that sometimes there can be an emotional link to an illness and having a treatment might release these emotions. If I was aware of this in advance, it would prepare me for any emotional release that she might have.

It was at this point that she informed me that a year ago she had contracted a virus that had attacked her liver. She fell into a coma, but fortunately for her the hospital was able to find her a donor organ and when she came out of the coma she was told that she had been given a liver transplant! A short time after the surgery she became depressed; her husband really couldn't understand this because the operation had saved her from certain death. Seeing her depressed had left him feeling confused and guilty because he had signed the papers for her to have the operation.

As soon as I heard this I decided to start the treatment because it seemed to me that Susan's physical health was fine but her emotions were creating an imbalance and I felt that I could do something about that. I asked her if I could do a mental and emotional treatment on her as this would enable me to use some of the Reiki symbols to target the depression head-on and this should make a difference to her health. She agreed and I began to scan her with my hands to see where the imbalance was being held. As I got to the area where the transplanted liver was, a surge of energy came from my palms and finger tips, it was very powerful.

Susan had told me that she was taking medication to prevent her body from rejecting the liver but she felt good physically and there had been very few post-operative complications with the transplanted organ apart from a little pain.

Now I knew why she had taken a huge amount of Reiki into the transplanted liver, it was because there was some emotional energy attached to it, this energy may have come from the donor as he or she may have been aware that their death was imminent.

As I drew the Reiki symbols over Susan's brow to start the emotional healing I felt her muscles relax and she quickly fell into a deep and peaceful sleep, and this continued right up to the end of the treatment. She simply lay there and slept like a baby.

I gently woke her after the treatment, she opened her eyes and gave me a smile; I knew that the treatment had done something because and as I looked into her eyes I could see the life force energy in them, they were sparkling.

Susan now proceeded to tell me that as she lay on the table, she felt a wave of energy pass through her body from her head to her feet and it gave her a warm feeling inside. This reminded her of when she was a little girl, when her mother tucked her up in bed just before she fell asleep and the memory of those times had made her feel loved and cared for. She had also seen a brilliant white light that seemed to fill her body, illuminating it on the inside like a giant light bulb. This made her feel 'tingly' all over but this hadn't frightened her; on the contrary, she said that it made her feel elated.

I asked her if she had felt any other sensations and she smiled and said that for the first time since the operation, the liver felt as if it was hers, in fact, she said that she couldn't feel the liver at all and this was unusual.

It appeared that Susan had now come to terms with her transplanted liver. She had accepted it emotionally and the energy that had been stored in it before the surgery had been released by the treatment.

The following day Susan and her husband came to see me and it was plain to see that she was a different woman. She was smiling, and that said it all.

Chapter 8

SOME RECENT INSIGHTS

I mentioned earlier in the book that Reiki is a great teacher and we may never fully understand how it works but as each day goes by I am able to reach a better understanding of its potential.

In the early years of my career, I practiced daily and thought that I knew what Reiki was, and how to give and get the best from this natural energy. Then one day I felt compelled to try something different. This was a huge step for me because previously I had thought that practicing Reiki was about repetition and that the more you practiced the basics, the better the treatments would be. Some of the Reiki books that I had read illustrated some different hand positions than the ones that I had been taught and the more books I read, the more confused I became! Eventually I realized that I was not meant to be a clone of Mikao Usui or any other teacher for that matter. I was given my individuality for a reason and I believe that this is to enable me to grow and develop. So now I decided to allow my free spirit some slack to see what would happen.

When I channelled Reiki now I moved to where I felt the energy was needed the most. There was very little structure involved in my decision making and on some occasions I made the right decisions, but at other times I wasn't so sure. I kept practicing and eventually it became clear to me that our intuition has a huge part to play when treating people with Reiki.

After a few weeks of 'informal' treatments, I started to experiment with different hand positions. I began to use just one hand for some of the placements instead of two and occasionally I would try using one or two fingers instead of the whole hand and what I discovered was fascinating. On almost every occasion that I did something different, the effects of the treatments were more powerful and the patients' response to these new hand positions was very positive!

One client told me after her treatment that when I placed my finger on her brow, it felt like something had penetrated deep inside her head. She said that she then felt something moving from inside her head and it travelled down her body and went out through her feet. I had placed my finger on her Brow because I *felt and sensed* that it was the right thing to do.

Listening to my intuition during the next few months helped me a great deal and it became the norm to do all of my treatment based on my inner feelings instead of repeating the hand placements that I had confined to memory. It is now almost impossible for me to treat a client in any other way because I am guided intuitively to where the imbalances are and I trust my feelings more than ever!

Most, if not all of the recent Reiki books state that Reiki energy is 'Spiritually Guided' but for the first time in my life I was experiencing some very powerful treatments based purely on my intuition and it felt so natural that I wondered why I had not done this before. I think I had been trying too hard and this meant that I was overlooking the obvious, that Reiki would guide and show me what to do, and where to do it.

In January 2009 I decided to book a holiday to Florida and while I was on line I found a Reiki web site which advertised books for sale. One book in particular caught my eye; the title was 'The Original Reiki Handbook of Dr Mikao Usui.' There was a brief description of the book and I thought that it would make a good addition to the Reiki books that I already had so I ordered it.

When the book arrived it was a revelation, because as I flicked through the pages, I found photographs of Mikao Usui's original hand positions and some of them were the ones that I had been doing intuitively myself before I had read the book, and this got me thinking! Did this mean that my intuition was being guided by Mikao Usui himself or other spiritual beings? Well, that could have been the case, but I believe that Usui sensei learnt *his* Reiki through diligent practice and because of that practice; he was guided to discover intuitively where to place his hands during his treatments. The other techniques he used were possibly a direct response to his knowledge of human anatomy and his innate awareness of his patient's needs. So, from this I deduce that there are even more Reiki developments yet to be discovered and this is an exciting prospect that I look forward to in the future.

Chapter 9

THE FINAL CHAPTER

I lived and worked in Cyprus for 6 years until September 2010 and every treatment that I did had fascinated and taught me something. Reiki is a therapy that is constantly changing and adapting to our needs.

I am aware that it is not possible to truly master Reiki because Reiki teaches us all there is to know, but only when we are ready for the experience. The Master/Teacher training class is merely the beginning and should not be the ultimate goal in the learning process.

Reiki was discovered and created for a purpose and I believe that this is to help mankind and every living thing that needs it, but understanding Reiki can be difficult. Numerous energies are at work, for instance, the energies within the treatment room and even the relationship between the client and practitioner. These energies are an integral part of who we are and can be felt and our awareness of these energies depends on our sensitivity to them.

THE AURA

Most of us have heard of the word Aura. The Aura consists of several layers and can sometimes be seen as moving light that surrounds the body. Many things can affect our energy fields including mobile phones, computers, televisions and electricity pylons and all of these objects can fragment and disrupt our electromagnetic energy. This in turn can have a detrimental effect on our health.

THE EMOTIONAL BODY

Our emotional body is a reflection of who we are. Our emotional experiences accumulate from when we are young and can have an adverse effect on our health. This is because we tend to develop problems based on what our emotions tell us, even though these emotions may not be relevant to our current situation. An example of this is the build-up of stress that can lead to many health problems.

THE MENTAL BODY

The mental body can extend beyond our physical body and is sometimes able to pick up vibrations from others by subtle perception or if we have psychic abilities. Our senses may detect this from buildings, people and other environments and the term 'in tune' is a good example of what we feel or sense. Our chakras are able to pick up what they need from a few feet away in the form of energy and this energy is then absorbed into our energy layers to balance us.

WHAT DOES THE FUTURE HOLD?

We have now entered another decade and we are all charged with having to recycle, conserve and create ways of living in harmony with the natural cycles of our planet. The majority of us have to rely on the energy companies for our fuel, unfortunately, very little of this fuel comes from renewable resources and it is being depleted at a rate that is not sustainable. Fortunately, Reiki comes from natural resources and is completely sustainable. This 'Universal life force energy' is available to us all and will never run out; it is a pure and positive energy that was created especially for our needs. Thank goodness that we cannot influence Reiki in a negative way as we have done in the past with our planet. This should be of great comfort to us all because as a species, we are very destructive. Since the birth of our planet, nature has provided us with opportunities to grow and evolve and as part of this continued growth, Reiki gives us the chance to give and receive from each other in a remarkable way. I feel that we now owe it to ourselves to 'grasp the nettle' and give kindness and comfort to those in need of our help. We have an incentive to do this because whatever we give out, we receive. If this is love, kindness and generosity, then what an amazing future we have.

If you are intrigued by what you have read in this book, then I have succeeded in opening your eyes to the possibilities that are available to you, however, please don't think that this book has all of the answers to the Reiki phenomenon. It is merely a glimpse into some of the wonderful opportunities that are available to you that will enrich your life.

A REAL LIFE EXPERIENCE WRITTEN BY ONE OF MY STUDENTS

My name is Zuzana Kristova and 2 years ago I did my Master-Teacher training with Philip my Reiki Master. Recently, Philip asked me if I would like to share one of my experiences with his readers because he had mentioned to me some time ago that a few of his clients had experienced something of a similar nature. I felt honoured to do this because Reiki has changed my life in so many ways.

I have to say that the Reiki energy that is channelled through me is very intense and the more I practice, the stronger the energy becomes. I have had many tremendous experiences that I would love to share with you but unfortunately there is not enough space for that, so I will share just one treatment with you that I did recently.

My friend George Agridiotis from Nicosia in Cyprus used to come to Paphos for me to treat him and during his treatments he would feel heat from my hands or see Angelic beings or colours etc. On this occasion the treatment was very different because something unbelievable happened!

I had just finished the treatment and as I was grounding his energy, I noticed that his legs were lifting up off the table, shortly after that, his hands, head and body lifted up in the air and the only part of his body that was touching the table was his stomach!

I knew that Angels and ascended Masters are sometimes present during a Reiki treatment so I silently asked them if they would settle him back onto the Reiki table when they felt that his treatment was over.

This unbelievable phenomenon lasted about 20 minutes and then as I looked on, his body slowly came back down to rest on the table. Shortly afterwards George began to cry and then he asked me how I had managed to make him float off the table! I said that I had not done it; I presumed that the Reiki Masters and Angels must have intervened at the end of the treatment for whatever reason. Both George and I were very surprised at what had happened, but I was grateful for the experience because it had given me an insight into a whole new world that I had not had access to before.

Since this treatment the experience has encouraged me to help and treat even more people.

Now I know that Reiki is truly amazing!

Testimonial 1

I was 28 years old and had been off the pill for nearly a year and had been letting nature take its course in trying for our first baby.

Being young I thought the road ahead would be an easy one. Nearly a year later and with no joy we could not understand why we were unable to conceive.

After trying and trying we finally decided to go to a fertility specialist to see if we had any underlying problems.

We were advised to keep trying for a further three months and if unsuccessful we would then start discussing options.

Three months later we returned with no good news and it was suggested that we try a drug called "Clomid" which is designed to produce more eggs to give us a better chance of conceiving. We went home and waited.

A month later, I was unwell and very low as I was in the throes of dealing with my father who had been in a riding accident a year earlier and had been in a coma ever since. I was very depressed and low and felt unable to take the Clomid.

I was having such a terrible time that when the next month finally arrived, I refused to take it.

A trip back to the doctor and after much discussion we all came to the conclusion that we would start the I.V.F. route in the coming August, it was now the end of April.

My husband and I decided that we needed a break to give ourselves a rest and to get some perspective so we headed off to Cyprus for a welcomed break and to celebrate his birthday. We arrived at the hotel and I headed straight to the Spa for some R&R. Flicking through the brochure I came across "Alternative Therapies" and 'REIKI' caught my eye. I had heard of Reiki as my sister in law had just completed her first diploma in it and had been told of its benefits.

I thought it would offer a chance to relax and break away for 90 minutes so I booked myself a treatment.

The next day was my husbands' birthday so we headed to the Spa for our treatments before dinner. I was greeted by Philip the Reiki Master; he explained the treatment to me and asked me how I was feeling in myself. I explained that I was extremely stressed and upset because of my father etc. but strangely failed to mention my inability to become pregnant.

At this point Philip asked me to lie down on the couch, close my eyes and relax, which I did. 90 minutes later I was gently awakened out of a light sleep by Philip who informed me that the treatment had finished. We sat and chatted about my treatment.

Philip asked me how I was feeling and I told him that I felt relaxed and energized; I then thanked him for his time and went off for dinner.

Three weeks later we found out I was pregnant, I can't even explain how thrilled we were, I couldn't believe it as we were meant to start I.V.F. treatments in two months.

We went to the doctors where my pregnancy was confirmed and was told my date of conception and would you believe it, it was the evening of my Reiki treatment.

I 100% believe that this was due to Philips amazing treatment, there was no way it could have been anything else. We welcomed our beautiful baby girl the following February.

We laugh and say that she's definitely a Reiki baby as she is calm and very content. We are very lucky.

Philip is an extremely gifted man, he is gentle and knowing and you will gain hugely by experiencing his incredible skill and gift.

I thank him every day.

TESTIMONIAL 2

"This is our Reiki baby story as we have lived it and even if it is a short chapter in this book it is the biggest chapter in our lives.

We must confess that we had never heard of Reiki before, but it came to mean a lot to us.

It was the most stressful time of my life when I was trying to get pregnant. I and my husband were trying many months before, but with no success. It was summer and we decided to go to relax at a hotel for a couple of days. Reading the spa treatments I had read about Reiki and I decided to try it. I needed so desperately to relax.

I was honoured to be treated by Philip, a person with many virtues. It was a magical time. As soon as the treatment was finished I felt the peace and calm in me. After the session I discussed this with Philip. I returned to the swimming pool where my husband was and it was a big surprise to him how calm and relaxed I looked. It had been ages since he last saw me like that.

I had another treatment the following day and something strange happened. I had a dream that I was saved and calm and could see bright colours and feeling of happiness and love. On those two days I got pregnant. We could not believe it. Deep inside, I knew that it was a Reiki child.

Soon after this, my husband expressed a wish to learn more about Reiki. He contacted Philip and arranged to attend a Reiki class. It was a fantastic day for my husband. He felt lovely and actually he mentioned to Philip that he felt a part of him was reborn. At the final part of the attunement when he had his eyes closed he could see different kinds of bright lights when suddenly they became darker as if blood was dripping. It was an unpleasant feeling at the beginning as it nearly went pitch black. But then the blood subsided and the light was back. He knew it was not the outside light changing because he had his eyes closed and his hands were over them. He mentioned this at the time but they didn't make anything of it.

My husband called me and I told him that I had a show of blood an hour ago. I could not go to the doctor as I was in another town and it was Sunday. That night as we were sleeping my husband had a most strange experience at the time. His hands were burning all night long. He woke up with the feeling. I was next to him and when he put his hands close to me they were getting warmer. He did not get much sleep that night but he was excited for this new experience that happened to him.

The next day we went to the doctor and thankfully there was not any problem with the pregnancy. Again we believe that Reiki's energy saved us. That was the only inconvenience throughout the pregnancy. I was calm and peaceful. I even had treatments during the pregnancy by Philip and my husband and this allowed the Reiki to flow into me and my child.

Children like Reiki and I wanted my child to have it. Thankfully I gave birth in the spring and our little child was born. She was a calm and relaxed baby, very observant, sociable, clever and of high spirit. She is the greatest happiness in our life and strongest energy force for both of us. One could say that it is genes that make her what she is but we are both certain that Reiki has played its part in giving us our baby and making her all that she is.

P & A Cyprus.

About the Author

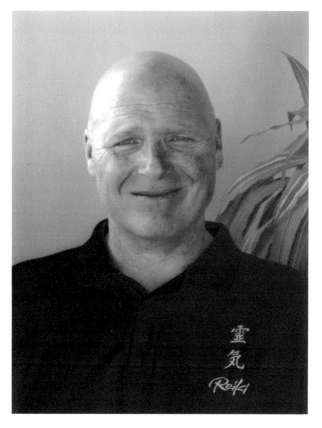

Philip Westwood worked for more than twenty years as a nature conservationist. His affinity with nature has had a great influence on many people over the years, his enthusiasm and passion is extraordinary and he has the ability to lift the spirits of anyone in his presence. He has been working for several years as a full time Reiki teacher and practitioner and has trained more than a hundred students, some to Master teacher level. His knowledge and experience is vast, due to the huge number of clients that he treated while living on the Mediterranean island of Cyprus.

His writing career started in Cyprus, with regular features in health and wellbeing magazines and this led to a number of articles being written about his work. Because he worked on a holiday island, there were people from all over the world living there and visiting the island as tourists and this gave him the opportunity to teach students from many different countries and nationalities.

Philip teaches a western form of Usui/Tibetan Reiki and is a member of the Guild of Holistic Therapists and now works in Cheltenham England in his own private practice.

A Reiki book like no other, this book will be invaluable for those searching for answers to how Reiki works and it will encourage and inspire you to want to experience the phenomenon of Reiki healing.

It is intended to expel some of the myths and misunderstandings that have been circulating about Reiki in the past and to open up new opportunities and experiences for novices, practitioners and teaching Masters alike. I sincerely hope that this will motivate those of you who have not yet tried a Reiki treatment or attunement to take the first step on this amazing journey of self-discovery.

This book is an account of the last six years in the life of Philip, a working Reiki Master. Philips treatments were witnessed by his clients and every case is factually correct and truthful and it is this that makes the book a fascinating read. You may find it difficult to believe the case studies that are featured in this publication, only time will tell and the true nature of what is possible will become evident from your own experiences in the future.

COMMENTS WRITTEN BY DAVID BADDEIL FOR THE TIMES HEALTH AND WELLBEING SUPPLEMENT

"The other treatment I had while in Cyprus was Reiki. The treatment was performed by Philip, a bald giant of a man from Smethwick. Philip simply held his huge Black Country hands over various blocked energy sites in my body and breathed deeply.

Now, Reiki may seem squarely at the quack end of New age practices, as virtually no touching is involved, but the fact is that as soon as Philip got going, I an insomniac, fell into a deep sleep, only waking myself up periodically by snoring."

TESTIMONIAL FROM A SPA CLIENT

"Flicking through the brochure I came across 'Alternative Therapies' and 'Reiki' caught my eye. I thought it would offer a chance to relax and break away for 90 minutes so I booked myself a treatment.

Three weeks later we found out I was pregnant! I couldn't believe it as we were meant to start I.V.F. treatments in two months."

TESTIMONIAL FROM A & P IN CYPRUS

"This is our Reiki baby story as we have lived it, and even if it is a short chapter in this book it is the biggest chapter in our life."

CPSIA information can be obtained
at www.ICGtesting.com
Printed in the USA
2472LVUK00004B